# PROPHYLACTIC AND
# OF GINGER AND GARLIC IN EXPERIMENTALLY
# INDUCED GASTRIC CANCER

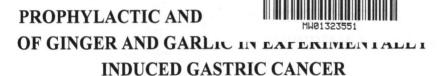

*By*
DEBJANI PAYOSWINI MANSINGH

## Copyright©2022

All rights reserved. No part of this publication may be reproduced, distributed, or transmitted in any form or by any means, including photocopying, recording, or other electronic or mechanical methods, without the prior written permission of the publisher, except in the case of brief quotations embodied in critical reviews and certain other noncommercial uses permitted by copyright law. For permission requests, write to the publisher, addressed "Attention: Permissions Coordinator, at the address below.

# CONTENTS

| Title | Page No. |
|---|---|

**CHAPTER 1: Introduction**

| | | |
|---|---|---|
| 1.1 | Gastric Cancer | 1 |
| 1.2 | History of Gastric Cancer | 2 |
| 1.3 | Incidence and Prevalence of Gastric Cancer | 3 |
| 1.4 | Etiology of Gastric Cancer | 4 |
| 1.5 | Signs and Symptoms of Gastric Cancer | 5 |
| 1.6 | Pathophysiology of Gastric Cancer | 6 |
| 1.7 | Diagnosis of Gastric Cancer | 7 |
| 1.8 | Management of Gastric Cancer | 9 |
| 1.9 | Garlic | 13 |
| | 1.9.1 Botanical Description of Garlic | 13 |
| | 1.9.2 Phytoconstituents in Garlic | 13 |
| | 1.9.3 Pharmacological Potential of Garlic | 14 |
| 1.10 | Ginger | 16 |
| | 1.10.1 Botanical Description of Ginger | 16 |
| | 1.10.2 Phytoconstituents in Ginger | 16 |
| | 1.10.3 Pharmacological Potential of Ginger | 17 |
| 1.11 | Need of the Study | 18 |
| 1.12 | Objectives of the Study | 20 |
| 1.13 | Scope of the Study | 20 |

**CHAPTER 2: *In-Silico* Analysis**

| | | |
|---|---|---|
| 2.1 | **Introduction** | 23 |
| 2.2 | **Materials and Methods** | 25 |

| Title | Page No. |
|---|---|
| 2.2.1 Protein Preparation | 26 |
| 2.2.2 Ligand Preparation | 27 |
| 2.2.3 Docking | 28 |
| **2.3 Results and Discussion** | 29 |
| 2.3.1 Interaction of Phytocompounds of Ginger and Garlic with Pro-Inflammatory Molecules NF-κB, COX-2 | 30 |
| 2.3.2 Interaction of Phytocompounds of Ginger and Garlic with Proapoptotic Molecules Bax and Antiapoptotic Molecule Bcl2 | 35 |
| **2.4 Conclusion** | 39 |

**CHAPTER 3: *In-Vitro* Studies on the Anticancer Potential of [6]-Gingerol and Alliin**

| | Page |
|---|---|
| **3.1 Introduction** | 40 |
| 3.1.1 Chemical Methods | 40 |
| 3.1.2 Isolated Organ Bath Studies | 41 |
| 3.1.3 Cell Culture Assays | 42 |
| **3.2 Materials and Methods** | 42 |
| 3.2.1 Plant Material and Preparation of Aqueous Extract of Ginger and Garlic | 42 |
| 3.2.2 Quantification of Bioactive Lead Compounds in Ginger and Garlic | 43 |
| 3.2.3 Antioxidant Capacity and Free Radical Scavenging Assay | 44 |
| 3.2.4 *In-Vitro* Anti-Inflammatory Potential by Cyclooxygenase (COX 2) Inhibitory Assay | 46 |
| 3.2.5 Evaluation of Anticancer Potential | 48 |
| 3.2.5.1 Cell Viability Assay | 49 |
| 3.2.5.2 Apoptosis Detection via Dual AO/EB Staining | 50 |
| 3.2.5.3 Wound Healing Assay | 50 |
| 3.2.5.4 Apoptosis Detection by Annexin-V Binding Assay | 51 |
| 3.2.5.5 Flow Cytometric Analysis for Cell Cycle Distribution | 52 |
| 3.2.5.6 Determination of Reactive Oxygen Species | 52 |
| 3.2.5.7 Measurement of Mitochondrial Membrane Potential | 53 |
| 3.2.5.8 Protein Extraction and Western Blot Analysis | 53 |

| Title | Page No. |
|---|---|

| | | | |
|---|---|---|---|
| | 3.2.6 | Combination Study to Check Drug Interaction | 54 |
| | 3.2.7 | Statistical Analysis | 55 |
| **3.3** | **Results and Discussion** | | 55 |
| | 3.3.1 | Plant Material and Extract | 55 |
| | 3.3.2 | Chromatographic Analysis of Ginger and Garlic | 55 |
| | 3.3.3 | *In-Vitro* Free Radical Scavenging Potential of Test Drugs | 56 |
| | | 3.3.3(a) *In-Vitro* DPPH Radical Scavenging Activity | 57 |
| | | 3.3.3(b) *In-Vitro* Lipid Peroxidation Inhibition Assay | 58 |
| | | 3.3.3(c) Ferric Reducing Antioxidant Power Assay | 58 |
| | 3.3.4 | *In-Vitro* Anti-Inflammatory Potential | 59 |
| | 3.3.5 | Cell Viability Potential-MTT Assay | 60 |
| | 3.3.6 | Apoptosis Detection by AO/EB Staining | 61 |
| | 3.3.7 | *In-Vitro* Scratch Assay | 62 |
| | 3.3.8 | Quantitative Analysis of Apoptotic Cells by Annexin V/PI Staining | 63 |
| | 3.3.9 | Flow Cytometric Analysis of Apoptosis and Cell Cycle Arrest | 64 |
| | 3.3.10 | Measurement of Intracellular Reactive Oxygen Species | 65 |
| | 3.3.11 | Measurement of Mitochondrial Membrane Potential | 66 |
| | 3.3.12 | Effects of [6]-Gingerol and Alliin on Apoptotic Proteins | 67 |
| | 3.3.13 | Combination Effect (Synergism) on AGS Cells | 69 |
| **3.4** | **Conclusion** | | 70 |

**CHAPTER 4: *In-Vivo* Studies on the Possible Mechanism of Action of the Test Drugs**

| | | | |
|---|---|---|---|
| **4.1** | **Introduction** | | 73 |
| | 4.1.1 | Rodent Xenograft Cancer Model | 74 |
| | 4.1.2 | Genetically Engineered Mouse Models of Cancer | 75 |
| | 4.1.3 | Chemically Induced Rodent Models of Cancer | 76 |
| | | 4.1.3(a) MNU-Induced Gastric Carcinogenesis | 77 |
| **4.2** | **Materials and Methods** | | 78 |
| | 4.2.1 | Induction of Gastric Cancer | 78 |
| | | 4.2.1.1 Experimental Animals | 78 |
| | | 4.2.1.2 Standardization of Induction of Gastric Cancer | 78 |

| Title | Page No. |
|---|---|
|     4.2.1.3 Experimental Protocol and Animal Grouping for Evaluation of Protection by Drug Treatment | 79 |
|   4.2.2 Measurement of Body Weight, Feed Intake and Water Intake of Experimental Animals | 80 |
|   4.2.3 Serum Biochemical Markers of Toxicity | 81 |
|     4.2.3.1 Estimation of Lactate Dehydrogenase | 81 |
|     4.2.3.2 Estimation of Alkaline Phosphatase | 81 |
|     4.2.3.3 Gamma Glutamyl Transferase | 82 |
|     4.2.3.4 Estimation of Serum Gastrin | 82 |
|     4.2.3.5 Estimation of C – Reactive Protein | 82 |
|   4.2.4 Tissue Collection and Processing of Tissue Homogenate for Biochemical Assays | 83 |
|     4.2.4.1 Assay of Glutathione Peroxidase | 83 |
|     4.2.4.2 Estimation of Catalase Activity | 84 |
|     4.2.4.3 Assay of Glutathione *S*-Transferase | 85 |
|     4.2.4.4 Assay of Glutathione Reductase | 85 |
|     4.2.4.5 Assay of Superoxide Dismutase | 86 |
|     4.2.4.6 Estimation of Thiobarbituric Acid Reactive Substances | 86 |
|     4.2.4.7 Ferrodoxin Reducing Antioxidant Power Assay | 87 |
|     4.2.4.8 Estimation of Reduced Glutathione | 88 |
|     4.2.4.9 Assay of Vitamin C | 88 |
|     4.2.4.10 Estimation of Total Protein | 89 |
|   4.2.5 Gene Expression Studies | 90 |
|     4.2.5.1 RNA Isolation and cDNA Synthesis | 90 |
|     4.2.5.2 Real Time PCR | 90 |
|       4.2.5.2a Estimation of Oxidative Stress Markers | 91 |
|       4.2.5.2b Estimation of Inflammatory Markers | 91 |
|   4.2.6 Protein Expression Studies by Western Blot | 92 |
|   4.2.7 Histopathological Analysis | 93 |
|   4.2.8 Statistical Analysis | 94 |
| **4.3 Results and Discussion** | 95 |
|   4.3.1 Standardization of Gastric Cancer Induction by MNU | 96 |

| Title | Page No. |
|---|---|
| 4.3.1.1 Tissue Biochemical Markers (LPO and GSH) | 96 |
| 4.3.1.2 Effect of MNU on Gastrin-Marker of Gastric Cancer | 98 |
| 4.3.1.3 Effect of MNU on Histopathological Changes of Gastric Mucosa | 99 |
| 4.3.2 Evaluation of Anticancer Potential of Test Drugs | 100 |
| 4.3.2.1 Measurement of Body Weight, Water and Feed Intake | 100 |
| 4.3.2.2 Protective Effect of Test Drugs on Biochemical Markers in Serum | 101 |
| 4.3.3 Anti-Oxidant Efficacy of Test Drugs | 103 |
| 4.3.3.1 Biochemical Markers of Oxidative Stress (TBARS, FRAP) | 103 |
| 4.3.3.2 Effect of Test Drugs on Enzymatic Antioxidants | 105 |
| 4.3.3.3 Effect of Test Drugs on Nonenzymatic Antioxidants | 111 |
| 4.3.3.4 Gene Expression of Oxidative Stress Markers | 114 |
| 4.3.4 Anti-Inflammatory Potential of Test Drugs | 115 |
| 4.3.4.1 Gene Expression of Inflammatory Markers | 115 |
| 4.3.5 Effect of Test Drugs on Apoptosis | 117 |
| 4.3.6 Histological Analysis | 119 |
| **4.4 Conclusion** | 120 |

**CHAPTER 5: Summary, Conclusion and Recommendation**

| | |
|---|---|
| **5.1 Summary** | 122 |
| **5.2 Conclusion** | 129 |
| **5.3 Recommendation** | 130 |

| | | |
|---|---|---|
| **BIBLIOGRAPHY** | | 132 |
| **ANNEXURE I** | Ethical Committee Clearance Certificate | 155 |
| **ANNEXURE II** | List of Publications | 156 |
| **ANNEXURE III** | Fellowships and Awards | 157 |
| **ANNEXURE IV** | Presentations in Conference and Seminars | 158 |
| **ANNEXURE V** | Publication | |

## LIST OF TABLES

| | Title | Page After |
|---|---|---|
| Table 1.1 | Role of Selected Spices in the Management of Cancer | 12 |
| Table 2.1 | Binding Energy and Docking Site of Selected Phytocompounds of Garlic with NF-kB | 31 |
| Table 2.2 | Binding Energy and Docking Site of Selected Phytocompounds of Ginger with NF-kB | 31 |
| Table 2.3 | Binding Energy and Docking Site of Selected Phytocompounds of Garlic with COX-2 | 34 |
| Table 2.4 | Binding Energy and Active Site of Selected Phytocompounds of Ginger with COX-2 | 34 |
| Table 2.5 | Binding Energy and Docking Site of Selected Phytocompounds of Garlic with Bax | 36 |
| Table 2.6 | Binding Energy and Docking Site of Selected Phytocompounds of Ginger with Bax | 37 |
| Table 2.7 | Binding Energy and Docking Site of Selected Phytocompounds of Garlic with Bcl2 | 37 |
| Table 2.8 | Binding Energy and Docking Site of Selected Phytocompounds of Ginger with Bcl2 | 38 |
| Table 3.1 | Quantification of Alliin from Garlic Extracts | 56 |
| Table 3.2 | Quantification of [6]-Gingerol from Ginger Extracts | 56 |
| Table 3.3(a) | Anti-Oxidant Capacity of Test Drugs – Scavenging of DPPH | 57 |
| Table 3.3(b) | Anti-Oxidant Capacity of Test Drugs–Inhibition of Lipid Peroxidation | 58 |
| Table 3.3(c) | Anti-Oxidant Capacity of Test Drugs– Ferric Reducing Antioxidant Power (FRAP) | 58 |
| Table 4(a) | Effect of Test Drugs on SOD, Catalase, GST, GPX and GR Level in Stomach Tissue | 110 |
| Table 4(b) | Effect of Test Drugs on SOD, Catalase, GST, GPX and GR Level in Liver Tissue | 110 |

## LIST OF FIGURES

| | Title | Page After |
|---|---|---|
| Fig 1.1 | Etiology of Gastric Cancer | 6 |
| Fig 1.2 | Signs and Symptoms of Gastric Cancer | 6 |
| Fig 1.3 | Description of Garlic | 14 |
| Fig 1.4 | Biomedical Properties of Garlic | 15 |
| Fig 1.5 | Description of Ginger | 17 |
| Fig 1.6 | Pharmacological Properties of Ginger | 18 |
| Fig 2.1 | Docking Poses of the Four Phytocompounds of Garlic with Proinflammatory Protein NF-kB | 31 |
| Fig 2.2 | Docking Poses of the Four Phytocompounds of Ginger with Proinflammatory Protein NF-kB | 31 |
| Fig 2.3 | Docking Poses of the Four Phytocompounds of Garlic and Diclofenac with Proinflammatory Protein COX-2 | 33 |
| Fig 2.4 | Docking Poses of the Four Phytocompounds of Ginger and Diclofenac with Proinflammatory Protein COX-2 | 34 |
| Fig 2.5 | Docking Poses of the Four Phytocompounds of Garlic with Proapoptotic Protein Bax | 36 |
| Fig 2.6 | Docking Poses of the Four Phytocompounds of Ginger with Proapoptotic Protein Bax | 37 |
| Fig 2.7 | Docking Poses of the Four Phytocompounds of Garlic with Anti-Apoptotic Protein Bcl2 | 38 |
| Fig 2.8 | Docking Poses of the Four Phytocompounds of Ginger with Anti-Apoptotic Protein Bcl2 | 38 |
| Fig 3.1 | Quantification of Alliin in Fresh and Dried Garlic Extract | 56 |
| Fig 3.2 | Quantification of [6]-Gingerol in Fresh and Dried Ginger Extract | 56 |
| Fig 3.3 | COX-2 Inhibition Assay of [6]-Gingerol and Alliin with Diclofenac | 59 |
| Fig 3.4 | Cytotoxic Effect of Test Drugs on AGS Cells | 60 |
| Fig 3.5 | Morphological Features of Apoptosis in AGS Cells Detected by AO/EB Staining | 61 |
| Fig 3.6(A) | Effect of [6]-Gingerol on Cellular Migration-Scratch assay | 62 |

| Titles | | Page After |
|---|---|---|
| Fig 3.6(B) | Effect of Alliin on Cellular Migration-Scratch assay | 62 |
| Fig 3.7 | Annexin V-FITC Assay for Detection of Apoptosis by Flow Cytometry | 63 |
| Fig 3.8 | Effect of [6]-Gingerol and Alliin on Cell Cycle Arrest in AGS Cells | 64 |
| Fig 3.9 | Detection of Reactive Oxygen Species (ROS) Generation | 65 |
| Fig 3.10 | Measurement of Mitochondrial Membrane Potential (MMP) | 66 |
| Fig 3.11(A) | Effect of [6]-Gingerol on the Expression of Apoptotic Proteins | 67 |
| Fig 3.11(B) | Effect of Alliin on the Expression of Apoptotic Proteins | 67 |
| Fig 3.12(A) | Combinatorial Effect to Check Drug Interaction ([6]-Gingerol and Alliin) | 70 |
| Fig 3.12(B) | Combinatorial Effect to Check Drug Interaction (Aqueous Ginger Extract and Garlic Extract) | 70 |
| Fig 4.1 | Experimental Protocol for Animal Study | 96 |
| Fig 4.2 | Effect of MNU on Gastric Cancer Induced Experimental animals | 98 |
| Fig 4.3 | Effect of Test Drugs on Different Physiological Parameters | 101 |
| Fig 4.4 | Effect of Test Drugs on Serum Biochemical Markers of Toxicity | 102 |
| Fig 4.5 | Effect of Test Drugs on Some Specific Markers of Gastric Cancer | 103 |
| Fig 4.6 | Effect of Test Drugs on Some Major Oxidative Stress Markers | 104 |
| Fig 4.7 | Effect of Test Drugs on Some Major Non-Enzymatic Antioxidants | 113 |
| Fig 4.8 | Modulatory Effect of Test Drugs on Thioredoxin and Glutaredoxin by Gene Expression Studies | 115 |
| Fig 4.9 | Modulatory Effect of Test Drugs on Some Major Pro-Inflammatory Markers of Stomach by RT-PCR | 116 |
| Fig 4.10 | Modulatory Effect of Test Drugs on Some Major Pro-Inflammatory Markers of Stomach by RT-PCR | 117 |
| Fig 4.11 | Effect of Test Drugs on Apoptotic Protein by Western Blotting | 118 |
| Fig 4.12 | Histopathological Changes of Gastric Mucosa in the Experimental Groups | 119 |
| Fig 4.13 | Possible Mechanism of Anticancer Potential of Ginger and Garlic Extract in Synergism. | 120 |

# LIST OF ABBREVIATIONS

| | | |
|---|---|---|
| AGS | - | Adeno Gastric Carcinoma Cells |
| ANOVA | - | Analysis of Variance |
| AO/EB | - | Acridine Orange/Ethidium Bromide |
| Bax | - | Bcl2 Associated X Protein |
| Bcl2 | - | B Cell Leukaemia-2 |
| BHT | - | Butyrated Hydroxyl Toluene |
| CAT | - | Catalase |
| Cat-D | - | Cathepsin-D |
| Cas-9 | - | Caspase-9 |
| Cas-3 | - | Caspase-9 |
| cDNA | - | Complementary DNA |
| CDNB | - | 2,4-Dinitrochlorobenzene |
| CRP | - | C-Reactive Protein |
| COX-2 | - | Cyclooxygenase-2 |
| DCF | - | Dichlorofluorescein |
| DCFH-DA | - | 2,7-Dichlorofluorescein Diacetate |
| DNPH | - | 2,4-Dinitrophenylhydrazine |
| DMEM | - | Dulbecco's Modified Eagle's Medium |
| DMSO | - | Dimethyl Sulfoxide |
| DPPH | - | 2,2'-Diphenyl-1-Picrylhydrazyl |
| DTT | - | Dithiothreitol |
| FITC | - | Fluorescein Isothiocyanate |
| EDTA | - | Ethylenediaminetetraacetic acid |
| EtBr | - | Ethidium Bromide |
| FITC | - | Fluorescein Isothiocyanate |
| 5-FU | - | Fluorouracil |
| FBS | - | Fetal Bovine Serum |
| FRAP | - | Ferric Reducing Antioxidant Power |
| $\gamma$-GT | - | Gamma Glutamyl transferase |

| | | |
|---|---|---|
| GSH | - | Glutathione |
| GR | - | Glutathione Reductase |
| GPx | - | Glutathione Peroxidase |
| GRx | - | Glutaredoxin |
| GST | - | Glutathione-S-Transferase |
| H & E | - | Haematoxylin and Eosin |
| HRP | - | Horse Radish Peroxidase |
| $H_2O_2$ | - | Hydrogen Peroxidase |
| IAEC | - | Institutional Animal Ethical Committee |
| IC50 | - | Inhibitory Concentration |
| IL-2 | - | Interleukin 2 |
| IL-6 | - | Interleukin 6 |
| IL-10 | - | Interleukin 10 |
| LDH | - | Lactate Dehydrogenase |
| LPO | - | Lipid Peroxidation |
| MTT | - | (4,5-Dimethylthiazol-2-yl)-2,5-Diphenyltetrazolium Bromide |
| MMP | - | Mitochondrial Membrane Potential |
| MNU | - | N-Nitroso-N-Methylurea |
| NAD | - | Nicotinamide Adenine Dinucleotide |
| NADPH | - | Nictotinamide Adenine Dinucleotide Phosphate |
| NBT | - | Nitroblue Tetrazolium |
| NCBI | - | National Centre for Biotechnology Information |
| NCCS | - | National Centre for Cell Science |
| NF-κB | - | Nuclear Factor kappa-Light-Chain-Enhancer of Activated B cells |
| NO | - | Nitric Oxide |
| NSAID | - | Non-Steroidal Anti-Inflammatory Drug |
| PDB | - | Protein Data Bank |
| p53 | - | Tumor Protein p53 |
| PAGE | - | Polyacrylamide Gel Electrophoresis |

| | | |
|---|---|---|
| PBS | - | Phosphate Buffer Saline |
| PGE2 | - | Prostagalndin 2 |
| PI | - | Propidium Iodide |
| PMS | - | Phenazine Methosulfate |
| PVD | - | Polyvinylidene Nifluoride |
| ROS | - | Reactive Oxygen Species |
| RT-PCR | - | Real-Time Polymerase Chain Reaction |
| SDS | - | Sodium Dodecyl Sulphate |
| SOD | - | Superoxide Dismutase |
| TBA | - | Thiobarbutaric Acid |
| TBARS- | - | Thiobarbituric Acid Reactive Substances |
| TCA | - | Trichloroacetic Acid |
| TNF-α | - | Tumor Necrosis Factor Alpha |
| TRx | - | Thioredoxin |
| WB | - | Western Blotting |

# ABSTRACT

Cancer is a dreaded disorder of abnormal cell growth leading to life threatening complications and if uncontrolled may also lead to death. Exploring nutraceuticals from plant materials to replace synthetic drugs and also to overcome their side effects has raised interest in recent times. Hence, in the present work two well-known spices *Zingiber officinale* (ginger) *and Alliium sativum* (garlic) which are also used in traditional medicine were studied for their anti-cancer effect on gastric cancer by *in silico, in vitro* and *in vivo* studies. To start with, the screening for bioactivity of four major phytocompounds from ginger ([6]-Gingerol, [10]-Gingerol, [8]-Shogal, Zingerone) and four from garlic (Alliin, Allicin, Diallydisulphide, S-allyl cysteine) were subjected to *in-silico* docking analysis using Autodock software on pro-inflammatory markers (NFkB, COX-2) and apoptotic markers (Bax and Bcl2). It was found that [6]-Gingerol showed pronounced activity in terms of docking score among other compounds in ginger whereas Alliin showed a potent docking score among all the other compounds in garlic. Considering the impressive results from *in-silico* analysis, [6]-Gingerol as well as Alliin was quantified in both fresh and dried ginger and garlic respectively. It was identified that [6]-Gingerol and Alliin content in fresh ginger and fresh garlic was more in comparison to dried ginger extract and dried garlic extract respectively.

Subsequently, the biological activity of both [6]-Gingerol and Alliin was carried out by *in-vitro* assays. As free radicals play a major role in most disease progression, the potency of all the extracts as well as the two bioactive molecules in scavenging the free radicals was evaluated by DPPH radical scavenging assay, Lipid peroxidation inhibitory assay and Ferric Reducing antioxidant potential followed by *in-vitro* anti-inflammatory potential by Cyclooxygenase-2 inhibitory assay. Further, the cytotoxic potential of the extracts and their bioactive compounds revealed that both [6]-Gingerol and Alliin exhibit potent cytotoxicity against AGS gastric carcinoma cells. To pin down the mechanism, morphological identification of cell death and cell cycle analysis using a flow cytometer revealed that [6]-Gingerol showed specific G2/M phase arrest while Alliin showed a growth arrest in S phase in AGS cells. Further investigation of phosphatidylserine externalization in AGS cells after the treatment with [6]-Gingerol as well as Alliin revealed the pronounced potency of both compounds in terms of apoptosis. The apoptotic effect was identified to be probably mediated by the loss of mitochondrial membrane potential in a time dependent manner through excessive generation of ROS in a dose dependent manner. Further, the mechanistic pathway by which [6]-Gingerol and Alliin induce apoptosis was confirmed by changes in the level of apoptosis-related proteins (Caspase 3, Caspase 9, Bcl2, Bax and Cytochrome c).

Ginger and garlic, the two commonly used spices in the Indian kitchen is used in combination in most of the recipes. This prompted us to check the combined effect of the aqueous extract of both ginger and garlic and the bioactive molecules [6]-Gingerol and Alliin. It is interesting to note that the drug interaction identified by compusyn software exhibited potent synergistic effect whereas the individual bioactive molecules exhibited moderate antagonistic effect. This clearly confirms the use of whole extracts and the synergism in most of the traditional medicine preparations. Based on the synergetic influence of ginger and garlic in modulating cell viability by *in vitro* assays, the prophylactic and therapeutic role of ginger and garlic in comparison to the individual extracts and the standard drug 5-FU was tested in MNU-induced gastric carcinoma in albino Wistar rats. According to the changes in the biochemical markers such as gastrin, LDH and ALP followed by oxidative stress markers in the stomach and liver it was identified that the combination of ginger and garlic extract is a potential therapeutic agent to suppress MNU-induced gastric cancer in experimental rats. The probable mode of action of the combination effect of ginger and garlic extracts in synergism was elucidated by some of the pro-inflammatory markers like NF-kB, TNF-α, IL-6, PGE2, COX-2 as well as by some oxidative stress markers such as Thioredoxin and Glutaredoxin in the stomach tissues of experimental animals by Real time PCR analysis. The mechanism by which the combination dose (prophylactic and therapeutic) induces apoptosis was confirmed by changes in the level of apoptosis-related proteins (Caspase 3, Cytochrome c, Bcl2 and Bax). Further, histological analysis confirmed the pathological changes in the experimental animals and substantiates the influence of test drug combination to suppress MNU-induced gastric cancer in experimental rats.

In conclusion, the results of the present work confirm that the combination dose of ginger and garlic exhibited potent anticancer potential modulating oxidative stress, inflammation and apoptosis both prophylactically and therapeutically. It also provides a new insight into the chemotherapeutic properties of ginger and garlic, which will allow the design of better management plans for gastric cancer patients.

# CHAPTER 1
## Introduction

# CHAPTER 1

**Introduction**

Cancer "The Emperor of all Maladies" is the most dreaded disease in the modern world. Aggravating stress levels, spasmodic sleeping patterns and contaminated foods with mutagens are some of the paramount reasons why cancer afflicts the chords of human body. Cancer is an agglomeration of heterogeneous diseases that differ in molecular and phenotypic characteristics observed by out of control cell growth, wherein specific tissues in the cells does not respond to the signals that control cell survival, proliferation, differentiation and death. In general, cancer disturbs cellular relations and results in the dysfunction of vital genes (Seto, Honma et al. 2010). A sequence of acquired or inherited mutations to distinct classes of genes which perform major roles in cell division, apoptosis and DNA repair is usually required for carcinogenesis (Dixon and Kopras 2004). Research showed that most of the cancer originates from the undesirable molecular, biochemical and cellular behaviors which leads to devastating outcomes.

## 1.1 Gastric Cancer

Gastric cancer is the most dangerous one among all types of cancer causing death in the world. In general, gastric cancer depends mainly on different environmental circumstances as well as the accumulation of specific genetic changes. This accumulation of genetic alterations is believed to be one of the reasons why it affects mostly older patients. The chances of gastric cancer increases with age and reaches its maximum at an age of 60-80 years (Pavithran, Doval et al. 2002). Development of gastric cancer can occur at both proximal and at distal region of the stomach. Globally, the occurrence of distal tumours is found mostly among people who belong to the lower socio-economic backgrounds. The major factors that lead to the development of distal tumours are dietary factors and *H*elicobacter *pylori* infection. The major preys for proximal tumours are the developed countries and its causative factors are gastro-oesophageal reflux disease and obesity. Intestinal and diffuse types are two forms of pathological variants found in gastric cancer. Intestinal metaplasia and dysplasia are the final outcomes progressive of intestinal type that originates from chronic gastritis leading to atrophic gastritis. However, diffuse type is linked with an adversarial scenario where the diagnosis is often delayed until the disease is quite advanced. This type is characterized by the development of linitis plastic (Hu, El Hajj et al. 2012). Intestinal type is more common among elderly men while the diffuse type has a more equal male-to-female ratio and more prevalent in individuals below the age of 50 (Crew and Neugut 2004).

## 1.2 History of Gastric Cancer

Until eighteenth century, there was little knowledge about gastric cancer. Only in 1835 for the first time J. Cruveilhier discovered benign and malignant gastric ulcers (Santoro 2005). Before anyone merely knows about this disease, scientific evidences confirmed that the death of Napoleon Bonaparte was due to peptic ulcer followed by gastric cancer (Hindmarsh and Corso 1998). In most of the Pacific countries like Japan, Korea, China and other countries, gastric cancer was a main death threat and most people died because of it for a century. Only after 2000s, these countries developed different clinical trials and treatments against this dreaded disease (Nakajima 2005). The first unsuccessful gastric cancer surgery was performed by Jules Emile Pean, on $9^{th}$ of April, 1879 while Theodor Billroth was successful to perform a surgery to gastroduodenal anastomosis in Vienna on $22^{nd}$ of January, 1881. Until now, millions of patients have suffered from it and undergone surgery (Yoshino 2000).

## 1.3 Incidence and Prevalence of Gastric Cancer

Till 1990s, main cause for cancer-related death was the gastric cancer. Despite a decline in mortality, it is among the five most dangerous cause for death throughout the world. Mostly people from Eastern Europe, Central and South America and East Asia used to suffer from it (Brenner, Rothenbacher et al. 2009). Approximately 6.8% of the total cancer cases were diagnosed as gastric cancer (952,000 cases, GLOBOCAN 2012, http://globocan.iarc.fr/old/FactSheets/cancers/stomach-new.asp). After lung, breast, colorectum and prostate cancers, most of the patients die because of gastric cancer. The estimated rate of this cancer is at peak in East Asia (0.024% in men, 0.0098% women) and bottom most in Northern America (0.0028% in men, 0.0015% in women).

In India, the rate of gastric cancer is low as compared to other developing countries but there are some areas like the Southern part and North-eastern states where the incidence is higher than other high-incidence prone areas of the world. In India, the highest incidence of this cancer is reported in Mizoram (30% including all cancer-caused deaths). Development of gastric cancer depends mainly upon food habit, food hygiene, sanitation, food preservation techniques, age group and gender. Men are more prone to it than women and their ratio was estimated as 2.3:1. The use of tobacco and alcohol also potentiates the chance of gastric cancer. In a case–control study from Trivandrum, eating rice and chilly in higher rate and consumption of high-temperature food were also found to be a cause for it (Mathew, Gangadharan et al. 2000). In comparison to males from Northern part of India, Southern part males are the main victim of it because of regional variations and their eating habits. Also in a study from Hyderabad it was reported that smokers ($P < 0.01$) and drinkers ($P < 0.05$) have more chances of gastric cancer occurrence (Sharma and Radhakrishnan 2011).

## 1.4 Etiology of Gastric Cancer

Different reason like dietary factors, pathological factors, physical factors, genetic factors, environmental factors and reproductive factors are associated with gastric cancer. According to epidemiological data, gastric cancer occurs more in males than females (Kelley and Duggan 2003) because women have estrogen which might be the reason for the slow cancer development (Qin, Liu et al. 2014).

The development of gastric cancer solely depends on the infection with *Helicobacter pylori*. As per epidemiological statistics from Asia, a person with *Helicobacter pylori* infection has more chances of gastric cancer than a person with no infection. Mostly, a person with age less than 30 has high chances of gastric cancer (Uemura, Okamoto et al. 2001). Smoking directly leads to intestinal cancer of the distal stomach. As per the systematic epidemiological analysis from Japan, a person who smokes has high relative risk of gastric cancer 1·56 (95% CI 1·36–1·80) than who does not smoke (Leung, Wu et al. 2008). Gastric lesion and cancer occurs in the upper part of the stomach near the oesophagus of a smoker (Pelucchi, Lunet et al. 2015). However, there is no sufficient proof that gastric cancer occurs in drinkers. In Korea, a population-based cohort study suggests that a person drinking alcohol (15 g/day) has 1·2 (95% CI 1·0-1·3) chances of distal stomach cancer compared with non-drinkers (Sung, Choi et al. 2007). Apart from this eating habits have a vital role in the development of gastric cancer. Besides, smokers and drinkers, a person with even low intake of vegetables and fruits develop the risk of gastric cancer due to imbalance in antioxidant and pro-oxidants.

A high intake of smoked or salted foodstuffs increases the chances of gastric cancer (Shikata, Kiyohara et al. 2006). People of South India are also prone for gastric cancer due to the high intake of chili and spicy foods in the diet in comparison to North India (Misra, Pandey et al. 2014). Around 1-3% out of 10% of family related gastric cancer cases, are based on genetic syndromes and are known as HDGC (hereditary diffuse gastric cancer). A defect of the CDH1 gene, lies on the 16$^{th}$ chromosome which codes for E-cadherin leads to hereditary diffuse gastric cancer (HDGC). Nitrosamines, that are carcinogenic for humans, can also cause gastric cancer in a wide variety of animals (Petrova, Schecterson et al. 2016). A positive link between nitrosamine and nitrite, meat and processed meat, fresh fish and preserved fish, vegetables and smoked food intake are supported by both oesophageal cancer and gastric cancer (González, Jakszyn et al. 2006, Jakszyn and González 2006). Most importantly, processed meat which contains $N$-nitroso compounds (NOCs) are high risk for stomach ulcer which leads to stomach cancer. Fig 1.1 represents some of the etiological factors related to gastric cancer.

## 1.5 Signs and Symptoms of Gastric Cancer

The symptoms of gastric cancer are abdominal distension, nausea, vomiting, dyspnea, and lower extremity edema (Saif, Siddiqui et al. 2009). Patients also suffer from anorexia, a sort of eating disorder, losing weight (95%) as well as abdominal pain because of large tumors blocking the gastrointestinal lumen or infiltrative scratches that damage abdominal expansion. Haematemesis, melena, or massive upper gastrointestinal hemorrhage happens because of bleeding in ulcerated tumors (Dicken, Bigam et al. 2005). The early stage signs are not specific and sometimes treated as peptic ulcer.

Dyspepsia happens because of one or more symptoms at a time (ex. burning, postprandial fullness or early satiation) (Harmon and Peura 2010) and most importantly weight loss, dysphasia and anemia. Many patients have the characteristic signs of heartburn or acid regurgitation and gastro-esophageal reflux disease. These are also termed as burping, abdominal rumblings, indigestion causing bad breath, ache in epigastria or felling uneasiness in the upper abdomen (Shaw, Talley et al. 2001, Talley, Verlinden et al. 2001).

Late complications of gastric cancer may include several symptoms. In some cases, palpable abdominal mass, cachexia, bowel obstruction, and hepatomegaly, pathologic peritoneal and pleural effusions are seen along with advanced tumors (Kim, Hyung et al. 2010) (Oda, Gotoda et al. 2005). Other symptoms such as obstruction of the gastric outlet, gastro esophageal junction or small bowel may concur to cause an increase in intra-luminal pressure which finally leads to ischemia (Salinas, Georgiev et al. 2014). Some marked signs and symptoms regarding gastric cancer are depicted in Fig 1.2.

## 1.6 Pathophysiology of Gastric Cancer

Environmental factors such as *Helicobacter pylori* infection and genetic susceptibility leads to pathogenesis of gastric cancer. Chromosomal instability, changes in epigenetic profile, somatic gene mutations or functional single nucleotide polymorphisms are the observed major genetic changes (Johnson *et al.*, 2014). As gastric cancer slowly develops over years there is a change in the physiological processes. These changes could manifest in different ways which involves an avalanche of precancerous lesions ultimately leading to invasive gastric carcinoma. Chronic inflammation is considered as the cardinal recognizable histologic change in this process and presented as acute gastritis, chronic gastritis and atrophic gastritis. Atrophy, is a form of mucous metaplasia and also known as spasmolytic polypeptide-expressing metaplasia (SPEM) and are presented in the gastric tissue either as multifocal or a diffuse pattern. SPEM is more strongly associated with gastric cancer than intestinal metaplasia and the probable precursor to the cancerous lesions (Halldórsdóttir, Sigurdardóttir et al. 2003). Therefore, gastric atrophy is a better sign for gastric cancer risk than intestinal metaplasia. In acute gastritis,

**Fig 1.1 Etiology of Gastric Cancer**

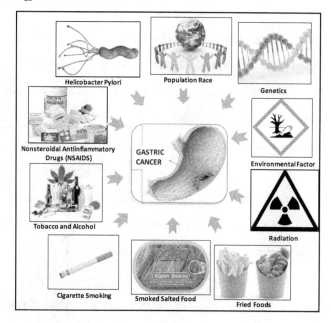

**Fig 1.2 Signs and Symptoms of Gastric Cancer**

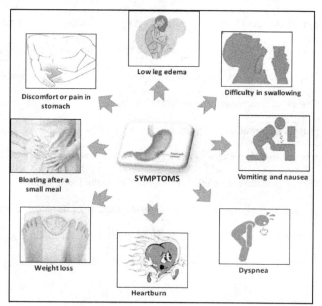

infiltration of mucosal and submucosal lymphocytes with pockets of polymorphonuclear cells occurs which is accompanied by mild mucosal defects and edema. However, chronic gastritis is characterized by moderate to severe inflammation along with marked epithelial defects like gland dilatation and mineralization (Fox and Wang 2007). The salient features of atrophic gastritis include chronic inflammation with focal fibrosis and complete loss of oxyntic parietal and chief cells. These sets of events are followed by intestinal metaplasia and dysplasia. Intestinal metaplasia is characterized by columnar elongation, formation of goblet cells, and mixed acidic and neutral mucins productions. The distinctive features of dysplasia are portrayed by in-folding, branching of cells with support from cell and marked cellular and nuclear atypia. Invasive carcinoma which is recognized as the final step accomplice with events such as: intramucosal invasion, degradation of the intercellular matrix and gastric intraepithelial neoplasia.

## 1.7 Diagnosis of Gastric Cancer

The early stage diagnosis of gastric cancer is often a cumbersome task as up to 80% of patient does not experience any sort of symptoms (Koh and Wang 2002). Majorly there are three techniques for diagnosis of gastric cancer. They are categorized as Endoscopic techniques, Imaging techniques and Molecular techniques.

**Endoscopic techniques** include Upper gastrointestinal endoscopy, Endoscopic ultrasound and Biopsy. Endoscopy which allows diagnosis of upper gastrointestinal diseases with a luminal or mucosal location allows visual detection of luminal anatomy which helps to determine the possibility of infection, and recognizes possible ulceration or bleeding (Sharma, Ardila-Gatas et al. 2016). Upper GI endoscopy is a frequently performed endoscopic procedure that is particularly suited for the diagnosis of esophageal gastric, upper small intestinal disorders and upper GI diseases (Guilford 1990). In modern gastroenterology and abdominal surgery, endoscopic ultrasound has become an essential tool. Due to the combination of endoscopy with ultrasound to obtain images of the internal organs, it became the most potential innovation than other tools (Sharma, Ardila-Gatas et al. 2016). However, biopsy is the only one method to diagnose gastric cancer where a small tissue of the patient is enough for examination.

**Imaging techniques** encompass Computed Tomography (CT) scan, Magnetic Resonance Imaging (MRI) and Positron Emission Tomography (PET) scan. Particularly, for diagnosing gastrointestinal oncology, FDG-PET/CT scan is used, Additionally, with this technique, different stages of cancer and their response to treatment, and reappearance of cancer can be noticed (Gauthé, Richard-Molard et al. 2015) which in-turn can detect nodal diseases with precise accuracy. 18F-FDG PET/CT may help in surgical planning and identifying different gastric cancer histopathologies (Marcus and Subramaniam 2017). Presently, CT scan is the most demanding technique to detect different stages of cancer. However, to find more precise location of tracer uptake in cancer tissues, recently, CT scans are combined with PET (PET/CT) and are also used for attenuation and correction of images (Kwee and Kwee 2015). Recently, development of MRI is the most advanced feasible tool to detect gastric cancer. Due to high resolution and intrinsic strength, MRI has the potential to generate contrast in soft tissue, which helps to understand staging in gastric cancer (Choi, Joo et al. 2014).

**Molecular techniques** to detect gastric carcinoma related malignancies include Immunohistochemistry (IHC) and Fluorescent In Situ hybridization (FISH). IHC is the most efficient tool where one can easily identify the early growth of cancer tumor more precisely after analyzing tissue samples. It includes the best diagnostic antibody panels providing critical interpretation of stain results (Tuffaha, Guski et al. 2018). However, FISH technique enables to asses genomic biomarkers to more insight on tumour heterogeneity (Pestova, Koch et al. 2018). In addition, specific RNA targets like mRNA and miRNA in cells can be detected and analyzed by FISH. It can also detect circulating tumor cells and tissue samples in gastric cancer related complications.

### 1.8 Management of Gastric Cancer

In general, the prognosis and treatment of cancer depends on its different stages. That means really it is necessary to know whether cancer cells are in only the stomach or circulated to the lymph nodes or other places. Moreover, it is very important to priorly know the physical and mental health of the patient. The treatment is much easier when the cancer cells are diagnosed at an early stage. However, more often they are detected in their advanced conditions and hence less chance to be cured (Sano and Aiko 2011). A range of treatment modalities apply which includes surgery (curative and non-curative), chemotherapy, radiation therapy, targeted therapy, immunotherapy and natural therapy.

**Surgery** is the best solution for cancer and has more possibility for the patient to be cured. Depending on the stages of cancer, different surgical techniques are generally adopted. Especially, endoscopic mucosal resection (EMR) is the best treatment method for early stage of gastric cancer, since in this stage mucosa only contains the tumor cells (Orditura, Galizia et al. 2014). The intention of surgery is to remove all grossly visible tumor tissue as much as possible which is in the range of histological risk assessment.

**Chemotherapy** is another way to kill or suppress the cancer cells. In this treatment method, patients are advised to use drugs to kill the cancer cells. The drugs also suppress the growth as well division of cancer cells. Most commonly, the drugs are orally ingested by a needle or in form of pill or capsule through an intravenous (IV) tube. The treatment via chemotherapy is always restricted to fixed number of cycles within a set time period (Wu and de Perrot 2017). The outcome of chemotherapy is to remove cancer related cells by surgery and reduce different symptoms that are developed during cancer. In some cases, chemotherapy is combined with radiation therapy. Generally, combination of two drugs such as cisplatin (Platinol) and fluorouracil (5-FU, Adrucil) are used for chemotherapy of stomach cancer. However, several side effects like tiredness, infection, vomiting, baldness, aversion, and loose motion cannot be avoided (Burstein 2000). These side effects are person specific and depend on the amount of dose used.

**Radiation therapy** or radiotherapy is an alternative tool to kill/suppress the cancer cells. It uses high-energy radiations, mainly X-rays or other radiations to damage the cancer cells or prevent their growth (Hallemeier and Haddock 2017), (Lewis, Chiang et al. 2017). This therapy is divided into two categories depending on the site of action: definitive therapy and adjuvant therapy. The former one is for locally advanced, unrespectable tumors and the later one is a surgery for high-risk disease.

**Immunotherapy** is another way for cancer treatment. This is also termed as biologic therapy. This type of therapy is to increase the immunity of the body or restore it to fight against cancer. This therapy uses chemical compounds those that are either self-made by body or prepared in the laboratory. (Niccolai, Taddei et al. 2015). Generally, many of the treatment modalities are combined for better efficiency and to increase the quality of life of a cancer patient.

In **targeted therapy**, specific cell, genes, proteins and tissue environments are targeted. The main aim is to stop the targeted cancer cell growth and minimize their effects on the surrounding tissue without any damage to healthy cells. Recent developments in targeted therapy includes identification of specific genes in a signaling pathway along with the factors involved in it (Yonesaka, Hirotani et al. 2016).

**Natural therapy** which consists of natural products or plant products, has shown potential ability to cure cancer with no side effects. Analysis says, thousand plants among 250000 plant species have the ability to cure cancer. In comparison to synthetic drugs that are used for cancer treatment, plant products are more effective to damage all types of cancer cells with minimal cytotoxicity. Plant products are also valuable in developing nutrient repletion to immunodeficiency people (Rajesh, Sankari et al. 2015). Diet including naturally occurring products or plant products are beneficial to health because they are non-toxic and in some cases controls programmed cell death in several tissues and organs. So understanding the mechanism of action of phytoconstituents might give more insight on their potential action (Chai, Shanmugam et al. 2016).

As gastric cancer remains an important and deadly cancer, studies indicate that person eating fresh fruits and green vegetables regularly lower the possibility of gastric cancer. These plant products generally rich with phenolic and organosulphur based compounds those play important role in the chemotherapy against cancer (Zhou, Zhuang et al. 2011). Since these plant products are plenty and are free from toxicity, their anticancer properties are widely explored. High intake of cruciferous vegetables like Brussel sprouts, cauliflower, cabbage and broccoli have shown to decrease the risk of colorectal, colon, prostate as well as bladder cancer in humans (Hecht 1999) (Lampe 1999, van Poppel, Verhoeven et al. 1999). Citrus fruits like orange, lemon, lime and grapefruit are rich in vitamin C, folate and fiber. Therefore, they play an important role in avoiding disease and maintain healthy life. Research on rat model signifies that grape juice containing phenolic derivatives are capable of inhibiting carcinogen-induced

DNA adduct formation and inhibits DNA synthesis in breast cancer (Singletary, Stansbury et al. 2003). For example, resveratrol, a polyphenolic compound inhibits ribonucleotide reductase as well as related cellular action linked with initiation, promotion and progression of carcinogenesis (Bråkenhielm, Cao et al. 2001).

Likewise, anti-proliferation effects of regular and decaffeinated coffee brews against ovarian cancer cell lines by inducing apoptosis are already explored (Roleira, Tavares-da-Silva et al. 2015). Polyphenols of green tea such as epicathechin, epigallocatechin gallate and cathechin decreased the risk of ovarian, breast, prostate, gastric, colorectal cancer and adult leukaemia to a tune of 40% (Shi and Schlegel 2012). Cocoa procyanidins have shown to exhibit potent antioxidant properties by reducing the concentration of reactive oxygen species and also have shown to inhibit LDL oxidation *in vitro* (Bearden, Pearson et al. 2000). Among many nonsteroidal anti-inflammatory inhibitors, turmeric is a powerful COX-2 inhibitor that has no side effects (Rao 2007). Off late there are a lot of manuscripts flooded in the scientific journals on chemopreventive action of curcumin and its analogues (Agrawal and Mishra 2010). Curcumin is the bioactive compound present in turmeric which has widely gained popularity among the scientific community for studying its mode of action in various disease conditions such as cancer, CAD, arthritis and immunity. Some of the selected spices and their anticancer properties are outlined in Table 1.1.

Ginger and Garlic are two spices that are not only used daily in kitchen but also as medicine owing to its anti-inflammatory, antioxidant and hypolipidemic activities (Gupta 2010). Since the present research work involves identification of the role of ginger and garlic on gastric cancer, herein we give a descriptive note on these two species.

## Table 1.1 Role of Selected Spices in the Management of Cancer

| SPICES | PHYTOCONSTITUENTS | ROLE | REFERENCES |
|---|---|---|---|
| *Cinnamomum verum* | Beta-caryophyllene, Linalool and methyl chavicol | Anticancer activity in leukemia and Melanoma cells | Mollazadeh *et al.*, 2016 <br> Azimi *et al.*, 2016 |
| *Syzygium aromaticum* | Gallotannic acid, eugenin, kaempferol, rhamnetin and methyl salicylate | Anti-inflammatory, Anti proliferative activity in lung and skin cancers | Rastogi *et al.*, 2016 <br> Perrone *et al.*, 2015 <br> Lee *et al.*, 2016 <br> Chanudom *et al.*, 2015 |
| *Trigonella foenum graecum* | Coumarin, phytic acid, nicotinic acid, scopoletin, fenugreekine | Anti-inflammatory and antitumor activity. | Sharma *et al.*, 2017 <br> Prema *et al.*, 2017 |
| *Piper nigrum* | Limonene, beta-pinene, Sabinene, alpha-pinene and hedycaryol | Reduces the risk of lung cancer by altering lipid peroxidation and by activation of antioxidative enzymes, Inhibits angiogenesis in cancer cells | Qiblawi *et al.*, 2015 <br> Zoheir *et al.*, 2014 |
| *Curcuma longa* | Curcumin (diferuloylmethane), turmerone, atlantone | Anticancer activity, Suppression of cyclooxygenase-2 (COX-2) and lipooxygenase expression | Li *et al.*, 2017 <br> Jiang *et al.*, 2017 |
| *Zingiber officinale* | [6]-gingerol, [8]-gingerol [10]-gingerol and [6]-shogoal. | Inhibits the production of free radicals, Suppression of angiogenesis in many cancers, Cytotoxicity activity in breast and cervical cancer | Abolaji *et al.*, 2017 <br> Kulczyński *et al.*, 2016 <br> Tzeng *et al.*, 2016 |
| *Allivum sativum* | Alliin, ajoene, diallyl disulphide, Alliicin | Antiplatelet, antithrombotic, anti-inflammatory property and in turn suppress cancer related malignancies | Khatua *et al.*, 2017 <br> Zeng *et al.*, 2017 |
| *Allium cepa* | Cepaenes, thiosulfinates, quercetin and campherol | Ability to suppress proliferation by retarding cell cycle progression and induces apoptosis | Ro *et al.*, 2015 <br> Nicastro *et al.*, 2015 |
| *Rosmarinus officinalis* | Rosaminic acid, apigenin, rosmarinic acid and diosmin | Increases the activity of superoxide dismutase (SOD) in inflammation | Rahbardar *et al.*, 2017 <br> Ghasemzadeh *et al.*, 2016 |

## 1.9 Garlic

Garlic (*Allium sativum*) is more commonly used as a herb in medicine and its medicinal properties are widely explored in literature. From centuries, it has been used as medicine to treat infections, heart disease, and cancer (Kaschula, Hunter et al. 2010).

### 1.9.1 Botanical Description of Garlic

Garlic is a monocot, bulb-forming perennial herb which belongs to the family Amaryllidaceae including two subspecies, ten important varieties, and hundreds of sub-varieties or cultivars. It belongs to bulbous plant group which grows up to a maximum height of 1.2 m (4 ft). Each clove of garlic bulbs is covered with a papery skin called as tunic. Each fleshy section of garlic bulb is generally covered with a crinkly skin. The plant produces leafless flower stem that are sterile producing bulbils than seeds. Such species are propagating clonally from cloves and bulbils.

The plant produces flower stem without leaf (a scape) and flower harvest only bulbils (small cloves) but not seed. Commonly, they are found in Central Asia and Northeastern Iran. It possesses a powerful aroma and a pungent taste and hence improves the flavor to the spice. It is also known as *Allium*, poor man's treacle, ajo, rustic treacle stinking rose, nectar of the gods, rocambole, camphor of the poor, and garlic clove (Adaki, Adaki et al. 2014). The morphology and taxonomical classification of garlic is shown in Fig 1.3(A).

### 1.9.2 Phytoconstituents in Garlic

Garlic has distinct nutritional profile with various bioactive components including phytochemicals such as flavonoids, fructans and phenolic acids. Garlic also contains sulphur-containing compounds: diallyl sulphate, alliin, ajoene, allicin (Craig and Beck 1999). The gastrointestinal health is maintained by fructans, small carbohydrate molecules by sustaining beneficial bacteria. In garlic, quercetin functions as an antioxidant which deactivates the molecules that causes injuries to cells. The flavor, aroma and potential benefits of garlic are due to its two classes of organosulfur compounds (γ–glutamylcysteines and cysteine sulfoxides) (Rasul Suleria, Sadiq Butt et al. 2012). Various bioactive phytocompounds present in garlic are schematically shown in Fig 1.3(B).

### 1.9.3 Pharmacological Potential of Garlic

The health benefits of garlic include cardioprotection, cancer chemo prevention, antihypertensive and cholesterol lowering properties. Importantly, cholesterol levels decrease (approximately 10%) upon consumption of 1 to 2 cloves of garlic per day. It has been observed that there is a decrease in cholesterol and fatty acid synthesis and cholesterol absorption (Koch and Lawson 1996). Garlic extract has also shown to have antithrombotic effect and it moderately decreases blood pressure (Hsing, Chokkalingam et al. 2002). Garlic has also several noteworthy effects and upon daily consumption, one can lower the blood pressure, prevent atherosclerosis, reduce the serum cholesterol and triglyceride levels inhibit the aggregation of platelets, and increase the activity of fibrinolysis (Chan, Yuen et al. 2013). Garlic compounds such as allicin, $S$-allyl cysteine have hypocholesterolemic, hypolipidemic and antihypertensive activity (Amagase, Petesch et al. 2001). Garlic is known to possess the property of preventing the generation of free radicals which helps in body defensive mechanisms (Amagase, Petesch et al. 2001). The serum total cholesterol and LDL cholesterol are significantly reduced upon garlic consumption. Garlic increases the HDL cholesterol moderately as compared to placebo in diabetic patients (Ashraf, Aamir et al. 2005). A significant decrease in glucose level were seen after chronic feeding of garlic extract (Banerjee and Maulik 2002). Volatile sulfur compounds of garlic such as diallyl disulfide, $S$-allyl cysteine, ajoene, and allyl mercaptan are

**Fig 1.3 Description of Garlic**

**(A)**

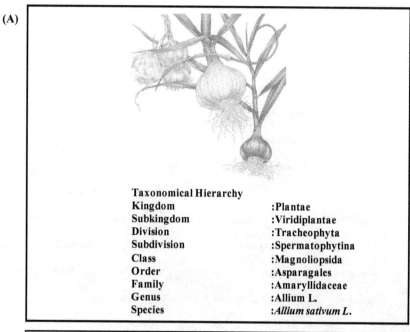

**(B)**

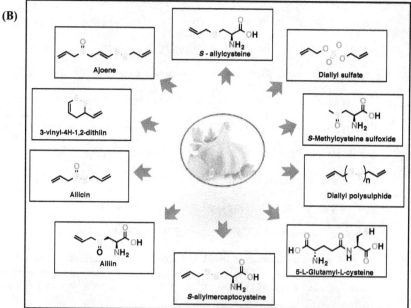

Note: (A): Morphology and scientific classification, (B): Different phytocompounds in garlic.

mainly responsible for protective efficacy against diabetes mellitus (Padiya and Banerjee 2013). Some *in vitro* study displayed the antibacterial effect of garlic extract against human dental plaque microbiota (Houshmand, Mahjour et al. 2013). The ethanolic extract of garlic also showed anti-bacterial activity against multi-drug resistant organisms which can be considered as a preventive agent in the treatment of microbial diseases associated with drug resistant pathogens (Karuppiah and Rajaram 2012). Garlic extracts also lower the uptake of oxygen, diminish different organism growth, stops lipid synthesis, proteins, and nucleic acids, and damage membranes (Bayan, Koulivand et al. 2014). The potent phytocompounds of garlic containing allylsulphide derivatives has been found to exhibit anticancer properties. The phytoconstituents of garlic such as diallyl disulphide, diallyl trisulphide, *S*-allylmercaptocysteine, and ajoene, can suppress proliferation of a wide variety of cancer cells by retarding cell cycle progression and inducing apoptosis. Some studies divulged that sulfur compounds that are present in garlic have apoptotic effect which was stimulated by increased intracellular production of reactive oxygen species (ROS). This proves the importance of the intracellular redox environment for induction of apoptosis (Nicastro, Ross et al. 2015). Some previous report revealed the suppression of cell growth of cancer cells by garlic extract is due to the cell cycle blockade in G2/M phase (Capasso 2013). Several components of garlic have also been found to possess anti-oxidative properties, stops covalent binding of carcinogens with DNA, enhance degradation of carcinogens, regulate cell proliferation, apoptosis, and immune responses (Tsubura, Lai et al. 2011). In liver, glutathione *S*-transferase activities are stimulated by diallyldisulphide and diallylsulphide, bioactive components of garlic (Munday and Munday 2001) by virtue of which it binds and detoxifies the potential carcinogens. Fig 1.4 illustrates the various biomedical properties of garlic in a pictorial manner.

**Fig 1.4 Biomedical Properties of Garlic**

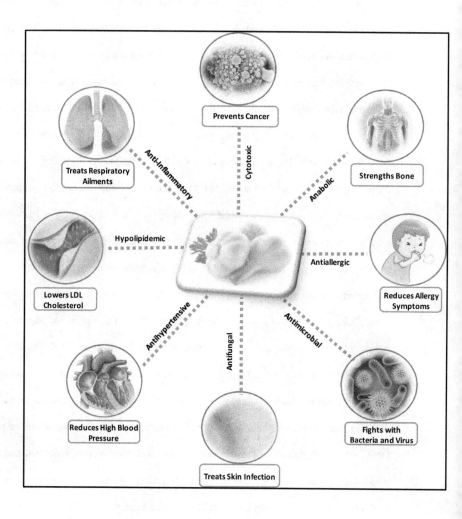

## 1.10 Ginger

Ginger (*Zingiber officinale*) is a widely-used spice globally and most popular in Asian countries. It is indigenous to Indo-Malayan region and has been cultivated in India since prehistoric times. The rhizome of ginger easily add flavor to foods and drinks and hence the use of sodium can be avoided. Presence of numerous bioactive phytoconstituents has made it to be used in ancient and modern medicine without any side effects.

### 1.10.1 Botanical Description of Ginger

Ginger is an herbaceous and slender perennial herb (30 to 100 cm tall) with leafy stems which belongs to the Zingiberaceae family and mostly grows annually in tropical countries. Generally, ginger plants are straight and contain fibrous roots, aerial shoots (pseudostem) with leaves, and the underground stem (rhizome) in which the rhizome has a corky outer layer which appears brown in colour and the center looks pale yellow and is used in cookeries and pastries. The underground ginger rhizome is much branched, somewhat resembling the palm of a hand with fingers which has circular scars representing the nodes with small scales. The flavor and pungency of ginger is because of some non-volatile phenol derivatives like gingerol, gingeridione and shogaol. Fig 1.5(A) portrays the morphology and taxonomical hierarchy of ginger.

### 1.10.2 Phytoconstituents in Ginger

50–70% of carbohydrates, 3–8% of lipids, terpenes, and phenol derivatives are the bunch of chemical constituents present in ginger. Phenolic compounds of ginger include gingerol, paradols, and shogaol while zingiberene, $\beta$-bisabolene, $\alpha$-farnesene, $\beta$-sesquiphellandrene, and $\alpha$-curcumene are known as the terpene components of this rhizome. Among the other phytochemicals, 23–25% gingerol and 18–25% shogaol are present in large amounts in ginger.

Ginger also contain protein, phytosterols, raw fiber, vitamins (e.g., nicotinic acid and vitamin A), amino acids, and minerals apart from the abundant phytochemicals (Grzanna, Lindmark et al. 2005). Zingiberene and bisabolene are considered as the aromatic constituents of ginger. Further it contains some compounds such as [6]-paradol, 1-dehydrogingerdione, [6]-gingerdione and [10]-gingerdione, [4]-gingerdiol, [6]-gingerdiol, [8]-gingerdiol, and [10]-gingerdiol, and diarylheptanoids. Presence of some pungent constituents like shogaols, gingerols and the mixture of the volatile oils in ginger are responsible for its distinctive odor and flavor (Shukla and Singh 2007). Various bioactive phytocompounds of ginger are enlisted in Fig 1.5(B).

### 1.10.3 Pharmacological Potential of Ginger

In traditional medicine ginger is used to treat vomiting, motion sickness, arthritis, cough and cold. Its antioxidative, antimicrobial and antifungal activity has been known for a long time. Nausea like sea sickness, morning sickness during pregnancy and chemotherapy can be prevented by consumption of ginger on daily basis (Marx *et al*, 2013). Additionally, rhizome of ginger that contains very high levels of total antioxidants (3.85 mmol/100 g), can combat oxidative stress associated with numerous diseases (Halvorsen, Holte et al. 2002). It has been proposed that, the ability of ginger to inhibit prostaglandin and leukotriene biosynthesis is due to its anti-inflammatory effect. During inflammation, [8]-gingerol inhibits cyclooxygenase-2 expression (Tjendraputra, Tran et al. 2001). Evidences suggest that ginger and its components have both *in vitro* and *ex vivo* anti-inflammatory effects. Studies have identified that aqueous extract of ginger has been known to possess anti-hypercholesterolemia effect in high-fat diet induced rats (ElRokh, Yassin et al. 2010). An earlier study proved that methanolic and ethanolic ginger extracts improved insulin sensitivity in gold thioglucose induced obese mice (Nammi, Sun et al. 2014). In herbal medicine practice, ginger rhizomes have been used for healing a

## Fig 1.5 Description of Ginger

(A)
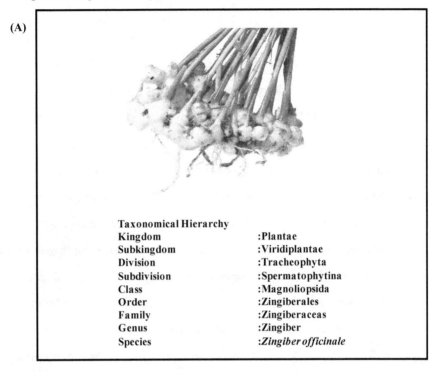

(B)
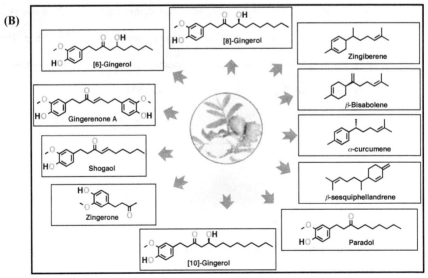

Note: (A): Morphology and taxonomical classification, (B): Various phytocompounds in ginger

number of diseases like rheumatoid arthritis, hypercholesterolemia, neurological diseases, asthma, stroke, constipation, diabetes (Lantz, Chen et al. 2007). Ethanolic extract of *Zingiber officinale* has been proved as a promising substance for its protective effects against cytotoxic conditions enforced by diabetes in pancreatic $\beta$-cells (Račková, Cupáková et al. 2013). Further it has been identified that aqueous extract of ginger influences tubulin and microtubulin stability. So, targeting the cytoskeleton proteins can be used as a major anti-cancer agent (Jordan, M. and L. Wilson 2004). The anticancer activities of ginger and its components can be explained by several mechanisms which include antioxidant activity, its ability for programmed cell death (apoptosis), decreased proliferation and cell cycle arrest. [6]-Gingerol appeared to be the most effective in inducing apoptosis in p53-mutant cells by causing cell cycle arrest, but not in p53-expressing cells (Park, Wen et al. 2006). Some *in-vitro* studies explained that anticancer activity of ginger is by up-regulation of caspase 9 and I$\kappa$B genes and down-regulation of KRAS, ERK, Akt, Bcl-xL, NF$\kappa$B (p65) genes modulated by mTOR, Wnt/ $\beta$-catenin and apoptosis signaling pathways (Tao, Li et al. 2018). The ginger extract has further shown to have anticancer properties towards ovarian cancer through p53 pathway in SKOV-3 cell line (Pashaei-Asl, Pashaei-Asl et al. 2017). [6]-Gingerol one of the major bioactive lead from ginger is also known to suppress cell growth by inducing apoptosis through G1 cell-cycle arrest in several colorectal cell lines like HCT116, SW480, HT29, LoVo, and Caco2 cells (Lee, Seo et al. 2008). Some biomedical properties of ginger are illustrated in Fig 1.6.

## 1.11 Need of the Study

Among all type of cancers, gastric cancer is the fifth most common cancer causing enormous number of cancer-related death. Its frequency varies greatly across different geographic locations and a major health burden worldwide. Adding to the burden, the diagnosis

**Fig 1.6 Pharmacological Properties of Ginger**

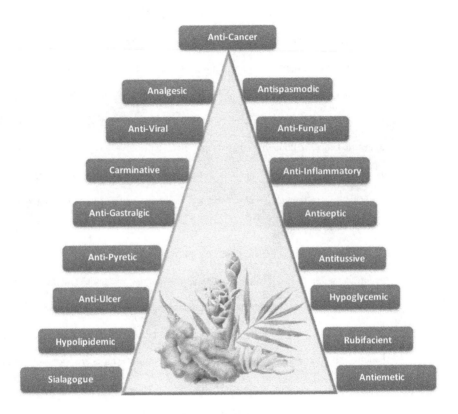

of gastric cancer is not easy and is identified only at the advanced end stage. However, prevention is the most promising strategy to control the disease. Smoking, drinking alcohol, genetic and certain food factors including *Helicobacter pylori*, causes gastric cancer. The present-day junk food consumed and style of living by people leads to high risk of gastric cancer. Most importantly, tobacco is a big threat and according to Cancer Research UK report, it leads to more cases in men (23%) than woman (15.6%). Besides, lack of fruits and vegetables intake, consumption of alcohol, overweight and obesity, excessive exposure to sun is also linked to gastric cancer. Although diagnostic and therapeutic advances have occurred during the past 10 years, there is no such advance treatment present to cure late-stage gastric cancer and conventional treatments like chemotherapy, radiation therapy and surgery have little effect on survival (Correa, Piazuelo et al. 2004).

Natural products such as spices are taken as a part of daily meal, as it has many beneficial properties to health. Besides anti-inflammatory, antirheumatic, hepatoprotective, nephroprotective, antimutagenic and anticancer activities, natural products also possess gastroprotective and anti-ulcer activities (Al Mofleh 2010). Therefore, exploration of novel beneficial properties of natural products and their scientific clues are necessary for the society. The knowledge can also bring new revolution in nutraceutical industries and health sectors. Although the Indian kitchen uses several spices in their daily cooking there is a dire need to identify the scientific basis of their use by Indians and the positive impact in the management of serious ailments.

Spices like ginger, garlic and its active phytocompounds are reported to inhibit the cell growth and promote apoptosis in several cancers like skin, colon, gastric, pancreatic and liver cancer which is suggested by the evidences from many *in vitro, in vivo* and epidemiological studies. These activities of ginger, garlic and their bioactive constituents may be inherent to the antioxidant, anti-inflammatory potential and other biological properties (Srinivasan 2014). However, there are no studies on the role of garlic, ginger and its combined effect to combat experimentally induced gastric cancer. Furthermore, the prophylactic and therapeutic potential of the combination and its mode of action in mitigating gastric cancer is unknown. Hence, prompts further study in these aspects.

**1.12 Objectives of the Study**

Based on the need of the study the present research work envisages the following objectives.

- To study the influence of spices (ginger and garlic) and their phytoconstituents in gastric cancer.
- To study the synergetic effect of the selected spices (ginger and garlic) in gastric cancer.
- To identify the probable mechanism of action of the selected spices (ginger and garlic) in MNU-induced gastric carcinogenesis.

**1.13 Scope of the Study**

In global scale, gastric cancer is considered as the primary cause of cancer death with respect to morbidity and mortality. Gastric cancer is caused due to *Helicobacter pylori* infection, diet or lifestyle, habits such as tobacco chewing and alcohol drinking or consumption of smoked/salty food (Dikshit, Mathur et al. 2011). The mortality rate of gastric cancer is high because it is most frequently discovered in the advanced stages. The common modalities of cancer management have their own side effects. Lately, researchers are focusing on treatment approaches which are effective with far lesser side effects in comparison to conventional drugs available for chemotherapy. At this juncture, the global pharmaceutical research has shifted their attention to bioactive molecules from natural resources to counteract metabolic disorders as they are accessible with a background of indigenous knowledge. Ginger (*Zingiber officinale*) as well Garlic (*Alliium sativum*) have been known to possess several medicinal properties like anticancer, anti-inflammatory, antibacterial anticoagulant activity. However, its role on experimentally induced gastric cancer in mitigating the pathophysiological changes such as oxidative stress, inflammation and apoptosis is sparingly known.

In the present study, use of *in-silico* technique to identify the potent bioactive molecules in the interested Indian spices - ginger and garlic would substantiate the role of the molecules on specific target proteins of inflammation and apoptosis. The study which focused on the specific objective would yield a proper scientific investigation and authentication of the use of Alliin from garlic and [6]-Gingerol from ginger in gastric cancer. Further, the *in-vitro* study would reveal the mode of action of the tested phytocompounds in grooming the organism towards eradication of an emerging tumor.

MNU a carcinogenic agent causes gastric cancer and several studies outlines different duration of inducing cancer. This study gives knowledge on the doses of MNU and the route of administration and duration of administration in inducing experimental gastric cancer in rats. The administration of MNU with 5% NaCl for 16 weeks and checking the intensity of the cancerous lesions i.e. 8 weeks and 16 weeks would give substantial evidence of the induction of cancer in the stomach of the experimental rats. The administration of test drugs (garlic, ginger and their combinations) after 16 weeks up to a period of 24 weeks would substantiate the role of these spices in alleviating the pathophysiological changes in the experimental rats with gastric cancer. Even more the study envisages in identifying the prophylactic as well as the therapeutic role of the combination of ginger and garlic in mitigating the pathophysiological changes such as oxidative stress, inflammation and apoptosis is worth studying.

The use of ginger garlic paste in most of the Indian cuisine reminds us of the fact that "Food is Medicine and Medicine is Food". The influence of ginger, garlic and their combination as an add-on therapy with existing chemotherapy would add value to translational medicine. This study yields a proper scientific investigation and authentication of use of ginger and garlic in gastric cancer. Furthermore, the outcomes of our investigation would prove the beneficial effect of garlic and ginger to lower the chance of cancer. The results of the present study will relieve people suffering with the anomalies of the gastric tissue such as ulcers and inflammation, the leading cause of gastric cancer.

# CHAPTER 2
## *In-Silico* Analysis

# CHAPTER 2

## 2.1 Introduction

Identifying a therapeutic measure which holds no inadequacies and acts reliably and definitely to curb cancer related malignancies is essential in the growing burden of cancer. Synthetic compounds such as antimetabolites, cytotoxic antibiotics and anti-microtubule agents are generally used for cancer chemotherapy (Chabner and Roberts Jr 2005). However, they injure the actively dividing normal cells also. As a result, administration of these agents to patients causes several side effects. Therefore, the necessity of novel chemotherapeutic agents from natural origin is the need of the hour to delay disease progression, increase survival of patients and improve tolerability. In the late 1980s, researchers planned to discover and develop anticancer agents that are free from several side effects and could able to target 'cancer-specific' molecules to eliminate cancer cells without affecting the normal cells (Sawyers 2004, Zimmermann, Lehar et al. 2007). Since these processes are time consuming, computational knowledge of drug design combined with chemical and biological experiments enhanced the drug design, development and their optimization. Computational technologies emerged as a pragmatic approach to curtail the gruesome experimental costs for screening of large number of compounds. Computational methods also help to realize certain molecular actions of the target macromolecule with candidate hits which in turn shepherds to the design of improved leads for the target by maneuvering the structural and functional information about the candidate. Virtual or *in silico* screening is the computational search for molecules in large computer databases with desired biological activities which can process millions of compounds per week. Owing to its effective property, it has gained superiority than traditional and even experimental high throughput screening (HTS). Virtual screening can be broadly classified into four types namely, ligand-based drug design (pharmacophore, a 3D spatial arrangement of chemical features essential for biological activity), structure-based drug design (drug-target docking), and quantitative structure–activity and quantitative structure–property relationship screening (Kapetanovic 2008). Structure based drug design provides necessary knowledge of X-ray crystallography, Nuclear Magnetic Resonance (NMR), 3D structure databases and active sites of the target protein and incorporates the target into a computer aided model. This helps in designing compounds that can bind to the target. Docking and molecular dynamics simulations are two commonly used techniques in this approach. Potent ligands can be found by screening a molecule database with docking software, while molecular dynamics determines the interaction between a molecule and the targeted protein. In addition, membrane permeability of the molecule can also be determined from molecular dynamics simulation (Lee, Huang et al. 2011).

Natural products which are the repository of structurally diversified bioactive compounds can be explored by molecular docking in an efficient and inexpensive manner and the involvement of molecular docking can accelerate and minimizes the cost of modern-day drug discovery process. A variety of modeling techniques are available for fast and easy analysis of suitable molecules against biomolecular targets. Among them, molecular docking is the best technique where the binding affinities of molecules can be expected by screening hits and affords structures with novel modes of binding. However, this technique is experienced as more difficult as compared to pharmacophore modeling but computationally most demanding approach, In drug design, selection of a target occurs by discovering one or more interactive molecules which can either promotes or inhibits the given target (Drews 2000). Conceptually, this will impact on successive reactions due to the concomitant changes in target protein activity leading to a significant development in the clinical outcomes. Due to the continuous improvement in power processing and capabilities of computer along with appropriate refinement of scoring algorithms, molecular docking emerges as a great promise in drug discovery (Ma, Chan et al. 2011).

## 2.2 Materials and Methods

Plant based drugs are proven to be potential owing to the numerous phytoconstituents present in them. However, only some of the phytoconstituents are bioactive and are known as active lead compounds for a target protein siphoning to an activity. Sometimes, two or three of these phytoconstituents may exacerbate its activity either synergistically or antagonistically. Ginger and garlic, the spices of interest in the present context possesses numerous phytoconstituents such as [6]-Gingerol, [8]-Shogal, [10]-Gingerol, Zingerone and Alliin, Allicin, Diallyl disulphide, *S*-allyl cysteine respectively. Gastric cancer is progressed by numerous etio pathologies such as oxidative stress, inflammation, apoptosis, autophagy etc. The underpinning pathologies can be targeted by drug molecules which possibly lead to the bioactivity. Identifying a specific lead molecule responsive for the anti-cancer activity was found worth pondering which further helped to narrow down the proposed research work.

Hence, in order to identify the influence of the different inflammatory markers (NF-kB, COX-2) as well as apoptotic markers (Bax, Bcl2) and its interaction with the bioactive components of ginger ([6]-Gingerol, [8]-Shogal, [10]-Gingerol, Zingerone) as well as major bioactive components present in garlic (Alliin, Allicin, Diallyl disulphide and *S*-allyl cysteine), virtual screening using bioinformatics tools was carried out to identify the best bioactive phytocompound before further studying their mechanistic role in inflammation and apoptosis related to gastric cancer. To carry out the *in-silico* docking analysis of the bioactive components from ginger and garlic with selective inflammatory markers (NF-kB, COX-2), apoptotic markers (Bax, Bcl2) bioinformatics tools like Autodock tools (ADT) v1.5.6, PyMOL Geowell iz3D, ACD/ ChemBiodrawUltra 13.0, ChemSketch (freeware version 11.00), Chimera 1.11.2 and LigPlot$^+$ were used.

### 2.2.1 Protein Preparation

Three-dimensional (3D) conformers of target proteins NF-kB (**4Q3J**), COX-2 (**5IKQ**), Bax (**2G5B**) and Bcl2 (**4IEH**) were downloaded from www.rcsb.org as Protein Data Bank (PDB) format for further *in-silico* docking analysis. PDB is a repository of 3-D structural database of enormous number of biological molecules like proteins and nucleic acids. The structures of such molecules are typically determined by either X-ray crystallography or NMR spectroscopy or both. PDB, especially structural genomics is one of the primary archival resources in areas of structural biology (Burley, Berman et al. 2018). Using PubMed (http://www.ncbi.nlm.nih.gov/pubmed), all the relevant literatures required for the present study were collected. This PDB database was developed by the National Centre for Biotechnology Information (NCBI) to provide access to citations from Biomedical Journals.

All protein structures were visualized in PYMOL to check for structural integrity and unwanted amino acid chains were removed to avoid overlapping results derived from homo, di / tri / tetramer proteins. Polar hydrogens were then added to the structure in Auto dock tools along with addition of Kollman charges. Atoms were further assigned as AD4 type and the PDB file was saved in .pdbqt format. PyMOL is a molecular visualization system that supports animations, high quality representations, crystallography and other common molecular graphic activities. PyMOL is a graphical user interface which is used to analyze molecules. Using

PyMOL tool one can visualize the molecule in any color and in any form like lines, sticks, cartoon etc. The H-bond and its length, distance between atoms, charges, and alignment of the proteins and the ligands can also be performed using this software. PyMOL was used to visualize the proteins by removing ligands from existing protein-ligand complex. The proteins such as NF-kB(4Q3J), COX-2(5IKQ), Bax(2G5B) and Bcl2(4IEH) were analyzed by checking the intactness of proteins and by removing the extra chains associated with the protein. Simultaneously, polar hydrogen bonds were added to the protein molecules along with Kollman charges. Then the proteins were assigned AD4 type atoms to strengthen the molecule. All the files were then saved in pdbqt format to prepare them for interacting with the ligands of interest.

### 2.2.2 Ligand Preparation

The bioactive phytocompounds of ginger ([10]-Gingerol, [6]-Gingerol, [8]-Shogal and Zingerone) as well as the major bioactive components present in garlic (Alliin, Allicin, Diallyl disulphide and *S*-allyl cysteine), were considered as ligands to carry out this study. This ligand preparation can be done in two different ways. Either the structure of ligand can be drawn on ChemBiodraw or it can be directly downloaded as 3D conformation from Pubchem as sdf format (https://pubchem.ncbi.nlm.nih.gov). UCSF Chimera includes a suite of tools for interactive analyses of sequences and structures, conformational ensembles, supramolecular assemblies and sequence alignments. Chimera is segmented into a core that provides basic services as well as visualization, and extensions to high-level functionality. In this context, after drawing the structures of ligands in ChemBioDraw, the 2D conformation of the ligands were subjected to 3D-optimisation by ChemSketch and converted to 3D conformer. Chemsketch is the best chemical drawing software. ACDLabs developed graphics tool to help chemists to draw molecular structures very easily, search reactions, prepare schematic diagrams, calculate all sort of properties, and design professional reports and presentations. Chimera software was used for converting ligand and protein files from .sdf to .pdb format. Ligands (.pdb) were opened in autodock tools and were saved in .pdbqt format after detecting the route.

### 2.2.3 Docking

Auto dock tools (ADT) v1.5.6 and Autodock v4.2 programs were used to carry out docking analysis (Sanner 1999). Auto dock is the most widely used and cited software and is also fast in providing high quality prediction of ligand confirmations. This gives an insight on how the small molecules such as substrates or drug candidates, bind to a receptor of known 3D structure. This software is also useful to find the location of the unknown binding site known as blind docking. To run Auto dock 1.5.6, a searching grid is generally used which was extended over the selected amino acids in the receptor protein along with the addition of polar hydrogens to the ligand moieties, atomic salvation parameters and assignment of Kollman charges. Gasteiger-type polar hydrogen charges were assigned and carbons are merged with the nonpolar hydrogens and the internal degrees of freedom and torsions were established. Thereafter, grid parameter files were saved in .gpf format followed by autogrid run. Computational binding or docking took place in between the bioactive molecules from the two selected spices garlic and ginger and the respective receptor proteins wherein the ligands were considered as flexible and the macromolecule was regarded as a rigid body. Lamarckian Genetic Algorithm was applied to carry out the search. The whole receptor protein was used for blind docking. Affinity maps for all the atom types present, as well as an electrostatic map were computed with a grid spacing of 0.375 Å. Search and docking parameters were selected before running the final auto dock. After accepting docking parameters, output files were saved as .dpf (docking parameter file) format followed by selection of program path name, parameter file and autodock was run. After completion of docking, the resulted files were saved as .dlg (docking log file) format. The final projection of the interaction and docking pose analysis was done by LigPlus, a software used to visualize the environment of a ligand either by downloading from the PDB ligand-protein complex or by extracting a docked pose from a docking run complexed with the target protein. To perform this, .dlg file was opened in auto dock and different docking pose conformation were analyzed using conformation play option in auto dock and hydrogen bonds were also build. The docked protein- ligand complex was then saved as .pdb format which was further analyzed using LigPlot$^+$ tool. Binding energies of different generated protein-ligand complex were also recorded by LigPlus. The final .pdb complex was run using LigPlus to show the active amino acid sites and hydrogen bonds between the protein and ligand. The results were evaluated by sorting the different complexes with respect to the predicted binding energy.

### 2.3 Results and Discussion

Inflammation and apoptosis are the major hallmarks of cancer pathology. Identifying specific targets to maneuver these pathologies would be ideal agents to manage the deadly disease. Hence, to find out the best bioactive lead to combat cancer, we have performed the *in-silico* docking analysis studies of different phytocompounds of ginger ([6]-Gingerol, [8]-Shogal, [10]-Gingerol, Zingerone) and garlic (Alliin, Allicin, *S*-allyl cysteine, Diallydisulphide) by targeting pro-inflammatory markers (NF-kB, Cyclooxygenase-2 (COX-2)) and apoptotic markers (Bax and Bcl2). The results obtained are analyzed and discussed with substantial reports in the present chapter.

## 2.3.1 Interaction of Phytocompounds of Ginger and Garlic with Pro-Inflammatory Molecules NF-κB, COX-2

There are meager studies on the role of natural bioactive leads from ginger and garlic on the inhibition of NF-κB and COX-2 in cancer chemotherapy. So, to choose the potent natural inhibitors of NF-κB and COX-2 in inflammation aggravated cancer, *in silico* analysis was performed with the four biomolecules of ginger and garlic respectively. NF-κB mediates a crosstalk between inflammation and cancer at multiple levels. In tumorous tissues with elevated NF-κB activity, the accumulation of pro-inflammatory cytokines at the tumor site directly contributes to the pro-tumorigenic microenvironment. NF-κB activity not only promotes tumor cell proliferation, suppresses apoptosis and attracts angiogenesis, but also induces epithelial mesenchymal transition, which facilitates distant metastasis (Mantovani, Allavena et al. 2008). Studies from *in vitro* and *in vivo* experiments have reported that down-regulation of NF-kB activity by natural and synthetic NF-kB inhibitors have been known to suppress the development of carcinogen-induced tumors by inhibiting the growth of cancer cells which in turn induces apoptosis (Sarkar and Li 2008).

The COX enzymes catalyze a key step in the conversion of arachidonate to $PGH_2$, the immediate substrate for a series of cell specific prostaglandin and thromboxane synthases which mediates numerous biologic processes. Various evidences collected from epidemiological, whole animal, and cellular studies indicate that unregulated COX-2 expression is a rate-limiting step in tumorigenesis and loss of regulation occurs early in carcinogenesis (Ferrandez, Prescott et al. 2003). Irregular up-regulation of COX-2 leads to pathophysiology of inflammation that finally causes human cancers. Since inflammation is a major process in advancement of tumor, compounds with potent anti-inflammatory activities are antedated to exert chemo preventive effects on carcinogenesis (Surh, Chun et al. 2001). Specific inhibition of COX-2 enzymes could theoretically avoid the gastrointestinal and other complications that are generally observed with the use of nonspecific COX inhibitors and therefore of general interest.

From the present *in-silico* docking analysis, it can be confirmed that Alliin showed a remarkably high docking score and interact strongly with amino acids of ligand binding domain towards NF-κB comparing with the other phytocompounds in garlic. The docking scores of NF-κB with different phytocompounds in garlic generated by autodock are included in Table 2.1 and the LigPlot representations of the best docked poses (Fig 2.1). From the binding energy values in Table 2.1, molecular docking studies revealed that Alliin exhibited relatively high interactions with NF-κB with a value of -4.463 kcal mol$^{-1}$ followed by *S*-allyl cysteine with a binding energy of -3.9 kcal mol$^{-1}$ while diallyl disulphide showed a value of -2.13 kcal mol$^{-1}$ and Allicin exhibitr a binding energy of -1.96 kcal mol$^{-1}$. As shown in Fig 2.1, OD2 atom of carbonyl group (C9=OD2) present in Asp239 formed H-bond with N1 of Alliin with a bond distance of 2.83 Å (A) while O1 atom of sulfinyl group (S1=O1) present in Allicin formed H-bond with NE2 of His141 with a bond distance of 2.87 Å (B), O atom of carbonyl group (C3=O2) present in *S*-allyl cysteine formed H-bond with N2 of Lys241 having a bond distance of 2.82 Å (C). However, diallyl disulphide showed only hydrophobic interactions with NF-κB and did not participate in any H-bonding interaction (D). From this study, it is revealed that Alliin, Allicin and *S*-allyl cysteine shared similar binding active sites with NF-κB which included similar amino acids like Tyr 57 and Lys 241.

Simultaneously, in the case of ginger, [6]-Gingerol exhibited good docking score with NF-κB in comparison to other three phytocompounds of ginger tested (Table 2.2). Probably, chemical environment of the ligand or different mechanism of action in [6]-Gingerol makes

**Fig 2.1 Docking Poses of the Four Phytocompounds of Garlic with Proinflammatory Protein NF-kB**

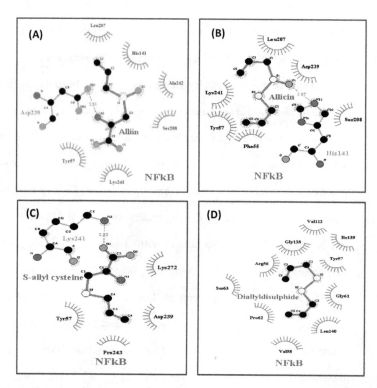

Ligplot representation of molecular docking analysis showing hydrogen bond interaction of NF-kB with Alliin(A), Allicin(B), S-allyl cysteine(C) and Diallyl disulphide(D).

**Table 2.1 Binding Energy and Docking site of Phytocompounds of Garlic (Alliin, Allicin, S-allyl cysteine and Diallyl disulphide) with NF-kB**

| S. No | Protein-Ligand Complex | Active Site (Amino Acids) | Hydrogen Bonds | Binding Energy (kcal mol$^{-1}$) |
|---|---|---|---|---|
| 1 | NF-kB-Alliin | Lys 241, Ser 208, His 141 | Asp 239 | -4.463 |
| 2 | NF-kB-Allicin | Tyr 57, Lys 241 | His 141 | -1.96 |
| 3 | NF-kB-S-allyl cysteine | Tyr 57, Cys 59, Arg 54 | Lys 241 | -3.9 |
| 4 | NF-kB-Diallyl disulphide | Gly 61, Arg 56 | - | -2.13 |

**Fig 2.2 Docking Poses of the Four Phytocompounds of Ginger with Proinflammatory Protein NF-kB**

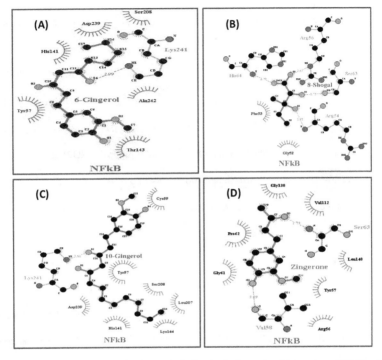

Ligplot representation of molecular docking analysis showing hydrogen bond interaction of NF-kB with [6]-Gingerol(A), [8]-Shogal(B), [10]-Gingerol(C) and Zingerone(D).

**Table 2.2 Binding Energy and Docking Site of Phytocompounds of Ginger ([6]-Gingerol, [8]-Shogal, [10]-Gingerol and Zingerone) with NF-kB**

| S. No | Protein-Ligand Complex | Active Site (Amino Acids) | Hydrogen Bonds | Binding Energy (kcal mol$^{-1}$) |
|---|---|---|---|---|
| 1 | NF-kB-[6]-Gingerol | Asp239, His141, Tyr57, Ser208 | Lys 241 | -3.55 |
| 2 | NF-kB-[8]-Shogal | Arg54, His64, Arg56 | Arg 54, Arg 56, Ser 63, His 64 | -3.45 |
| 3 | NF-kB-[10]-Gingerol | Leu207, His141, Tyr57, Ser208 | Lys 241 | -0.92 |
| 4 | NFkB-Zingerone | Pro62, Gly61, Val112, Arg56 | Val 58, Ser 63 | -3.54 |

significant interactions. The LigPlot representations of the best docked poses in ginger are shown in Fig 2.2. As shown, the O4 atom of carbonyl group (C12=O4) present in [6]-Gingerol formed H-bond with N2 of Lys241 with a bond length 2.99 Å (A) while [8]-Shogal formed four H-bonding interactions with four different amino acids (His64, Arg56, Ser63 and Arg54) (B). In detail, O3 and O4 atom of carboxylic acid group present in [8]-Shogal formed H-bond of distances 2.67 Å and 2.79 Å with NK of Arg56 and N atom of amine group present in His64 respectively. In addition, O2 atom of carbonyl group (C3=O2) and O1 atom of alkoxy group (C10-O2) present in [8]-Shogal formed H-bond of distances of 2.75 Å and 2.92 Å with OG atom of alkoxy group (CB-OG) present in Ser63 and N atom of amine group present in Arg54 respectively. In case of [10]-Gingerol (C), its O2 atom of carbonyl group (C10=O2) formed H-bond of length 2.61 Å with NZ atom of amine group present in Lys241 while Zingerone formed two H-bonding interactions with two different amino acids (Ser63 and Val58) (D). In detail, O atom carbonyl group (C=O) and O1 atom of hydroxyl group (C9-O1) present in Zingerone formed H-bonds of length 2.79 Å and 3.09 Å with N atom of amine group present in Ser63 and O atom of carbonyl group present in Val58 respectively.

From this study, it is revealed that [6]-Gingerol and [10]-Gingerol shared similar binding active sites like Tyr57, Ser208, Asp239 and His141 with NF-κB. [6]-Gingerol showed the highest binding energy of -3.55 kcal mol$^{-1}$ in comparison to the other three phytocompounds of ginger which further motivated to identify its role as an anticancer agent.

Like NF-kB, the interactions of different phytocompounds in garlic with COX-2 were explored. The docking scores of COX-2 with different phytocompounds in garlic generated by autodock are included in Table 2.3 and the LigPlot$^+$ representations of the best docked poses are shown in Fig 2.3. From Table 2.3, it was confirmed that, Alliin exhibited a relatively higher interaction with COX-2 with a value of -4.463 kcal mol$^{-1}$ and that was comparable with the standard COX-2 inhibitor (-4.7 kcal mol$^{-1}$) Diclofenac. In addition, COX-2 interacted with $S$-allyl cysteine and Allicin with a binding energy of -3.48 kcal mol$^{-1}$ -2.04 kcal mol$^{-1}$ respectively. However, a weak interaction between COX-2 and Diallyl disulphide was observed (-1.74 kcal mol$^{-1}$).

As shown in Fig 2.3 (A) the carboxylate-O atoms (O1 and O2) of diclofenac formed H-bonds of length 2.73 Å and 2.79 Å with OG atom of carbonyl group (CB=OG) present in Ser581 and imidazole-N of His351 respectively. In addition, N atom amine group present in His351 formed H-bond of length 3.03 Å with O atom of carbonyl group present in Asp347. However, Alliin formed three H-bonding interaction with three different amino acids (Glu484, Glu486 and Arg438) (B). In details, N1 atom of amine, O1 atom of carboxylate and O atom of sulfinyl (S=O) groups present in Alliin formed H-bonds of length 2.59 Å, 3.05 Å and 2.71 Å with O of carboxylate group present in Glu484, with O of carboxylate group present in Glu486 and amine-N of Arg438 respectively. As shown in Fig 2.3 (C), Allicin formed bifurcated H-bonding interaction with Lys186 and Arg185, where O1 atom of sulfinyl group (S1=O1) present in Allicin formed H-bonds of length 2.85 Å with amine-N of Lys186 and of 2.97 Å with amine-N of Arg185 respectively. Similarly, $S$-allyl cysteine created three H-bonding interactions with Lys180 and Glu176 (Fig 2.3(D)) where carboxylic group (O1 and O2) of $S$-allyl cysteine formed H-bonds of length 2.84 Å with carboxylate-O of Glu176 and 2.86 Å with amine-N of Lys180. In addition, amine-N1 of $S$-allyl cysteine formed H-bond of length 2.65 Å with carboxylate-O of Glu176 while diallyl disulphide did not show any H-bond interactions (Fig 2.3 (E)). Apart from this, it was also identified that except $S$-allyl cysteine, Alliin, Allicin and diallyl disulphide shared similar binding active sites like Gly 437, Arg 438, Ile 188, Gly 436.

**Fig 2.3 Docking Poses of the Four Phytocompounds of Garlic and Diclofenac with Proinflammatory Protein COX-2**

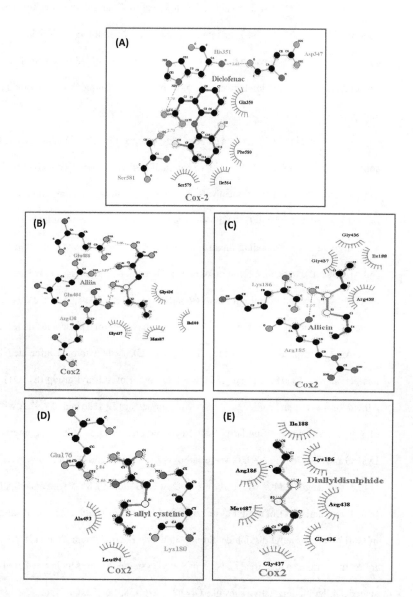

Ligplot representation of molecular docking analysis showing hydrogen bond interaction of COX-2 with Alliin(A), Allicin(B), S-allyl cysteine(C) and Diallyl disulphide(D)

In the case of ginger, the interaction of COX-2 with [6]-Gingerol, [8]-Shogal, [10]-Gingerol, and Zingerone, their respective binding energies and docking sites are shown in Table 2.4. From the molecular docking studies, it was predicted that COX-2 showed relatively high interactions with [6]-Gingerol (-3.55 kcal mol$^{-1}$) and Zingerone (-3.54 kcal mol$^{-1}$) than the other two. However, the observed highest binding energy was lower as compared to the binding energy of Diclofenac (-4.7 kcal mol$^{-1}$).

The docking poses of COX-2 with ligands diclofenac, [6]-Gingerol, [8]-Shogal, [10]-Gingerol, and Zingerone are shown in Fig 2.4. As shown in Fig 2.4 (A), similar H-bonding interactions between Diclofenac and two amino acids (His351 and Ser581) were observed as seen in the case of garlic (Fig 2.3 (A)). [6]-Gingerol formed two H-bonding interactions with Trp387 through its' O3 and O4 atoms of two carbonyl groups of distances 2.61 Å and 3.20 Å with amine-N and carbonyl-O atoms of Trp387 respectively (Fig 2.4(B)). As shown in Fig 2.4 (C), in case of [8]-Shogal, O1 atom of alkoxy group formed bifurcated H-bonding interactions of 2.50 Å and 2.97 Å with alkoxy-O1 and amine-N of Lys186. In addition, O3 atom of carboxylate group present in [8]-Shogal formed H-bond of length 2.88 Å with amine-N of Lys186. In the same time, O1 atom of carbonyl group (C6=O1) present in [10]-Gingerol formed H-bond of length 2.81 Å with carbonyl-O atom of Arg184 (Fig 2.4 (D)). However, Zingerone showed interesting tetrafurated H-bonding interactions with three different amino acids (Arg 438, Arg185 and Lys186) (Fig 2.4 (E)). In detail, O1 of hydroxyl group present in Zingerone formed H bond of lengths 2.50 Å, 2.90 Å, 2.64 Å and 2.74 Å with carbonyl-O of Arg438, amine-N of Arg185, carbonyl-O of Lys186 and amine-N of Lys 186 respectively. In addition, carbonyl-O atom of Zingerone formed H-bond of length 2.73 Å with amine-N of Arg438.

**Table 2.3 Binding Energy and Docking Site of Phytocompounds of Garlic (Alliin, Allicin, S-Allyl Cysteine and Diallyl Disulphide) with COX-2**

| S. No | Protein-Ligand Complex | Active Site (Amino Acids) | Hydrogen Bonds | Binding Energy (kcal mol$^{-1}$) |
|---|---|---|---|---|
| 1 | COX-2-Diclofenac | Gln 350, Ser 579, Phe 580, Ile 564 | Asp 347, His 351, Ser 581 | -4.7 |
| 2 | COX-2-Alliin | Lys 180, Arg 185, Glu 490 | Arg 438, Glu 484, Glu 486 | -4.463 |
| 3 | COX-2-Allicin | Arg 438, Glu 486, Lys 180 | Arg 185, Lys 186 | -2.04 |
| 4 | COX-2-S-allyl-cysteine | Arg 185, Glu 490, Lys180 | Glu 176, Lys 180 | -3.48 |
| 5 | COX-2-Diallyl-disulphide | Arg 185, Arg 438, Glu 490 | – | -1.74 |

**Table 2.4 Binding Energy and Active Site of Phytocompounds of Ginger ([6]-Gingerol, [8]-Shogal, [10]-Gingerol and Zingerone) with COX-2**

| S. No | Protein-Ligand Complex | Active Site (Amino Acids) | Hydrogen Bonds | Binding Energy (kcal mol$^{-1}$) |
|---|---|---|---|---|
| 1 | COX-2-diclofenac | Gln350, Ser579, Phe580, Ile564 | Asp347, His351, Ser581 | -4.7 |
| 2 | COX-2-[6]-Gingerol | Trp387, Ser530, Gly526 | Trp387 | -4.29 |
| 3 | COX-2-[8]-Shogal | Arg185, Lys180, Arg438 | Lys186 | -2.19 |
| 4 | COX-2-[10]-Gingerol | Glu490, Lys180, Arg185 | Arg184 | -0.74 |
| 5 | COX-2-Zingerone | Lys186, Arg185 | Arg185, Lys186, Arg438 | -3.44 |

**Fig 2.4 Docking Poses of the Four Phytocompounds of Ginger and Diclofenac with Proinflammatory Protein COX-2**

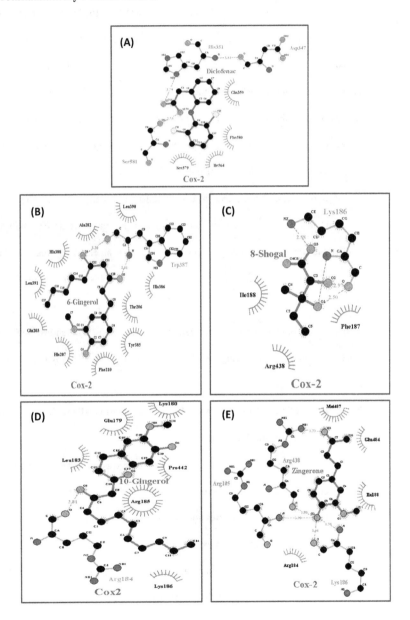

Ligplot representation of molecular docking analysis showing hydrogen bond interaction of COX-2 with [6]-Gingerol(A), [8]-Shogal(B), [10]-Gingerol(C) and Zingerone(D).

From the above results, it can be concluded that, [6]-Gingerol in ginger and Alliin in garlic exhibited higher interaction with NF-kB and COX-2 than the other phytocompounds tested. The cytosol of most of the cells express NF-kB wherein the inhibitory protein (I-kB) is activated and translocated to the nucleus where the regulation of more than 200 genes occur that helps in infection and cell growth (Kracht 2007). Numerous cancers and inflammatory disorders have been proved to be regulated by NF-kB signaling, by production of cytokines, inhibitors of apoptosis, MMPs for metastasis of tumor cells (Makarov 2000). Thus, targeting transcription factor, NF-κB can be considered as a novel preventive and therapeutic target molecule in the design of anti-inflammatory and pro-apoptotic drugs. Inhibition, of NF-κB pathway in cancer chemotherapy is now developing as an emerging treatment identified in the present study. Moreover, it can be assumed that natural NF-κB and COX-2 inhibitors enhance the effects of conventional cancer therapeutics, suggesting that down-regulation of NF-κB as well COX-2 could sensitize cancer cells to conventional therapeutics. Such approaches can offer the promise of enhancing the efficacy of cancer chemotherapy (Yamamoto and Gaynor 2001).

### 2.3.2 Interaction of Phytocompounds of Ginger and Garlic with Proapoptotic Molecule Bax and Antiapoptotic Molecule Bcl2

It has been reported that expression of Bax was associated with better prognosis in gastric cancer. Bcl2 can be considered a "generalized cell death suppressor gene" and as an inhibitor of apoptosis. Bcl2 expression is a potential mechanism by which tumor cells escape p53-mediated apoptosis and their expression has been reported for a variety of human epithelial malignant tumors, including stomach and colon carcinomas (Forones, Carvalho et al. 2005). Aizawa and coworkers showed that in advanced gastric cancer the expression of Bcl2 was associated with a lower apoptotic index and a better prognosis. Hence, the role of Bax and Bcl2, the proapoptotic molecules were checked for its possible interaction with the phytocompounds of garlic as well as ginger and discussed.

In silico docking analysis of garlic phytocompounds with proapoptotic molecule Bax were undertaken and results are shown in Table 2.5. The corresponding LigPlot$^+$ representations of the best docked poses are shown in Fig 2.5. From Table 2.5, molecular docking studies anticipated that S-allyl cysteine exhibited highest interactions with Bax with a binding energy of -1.94 kcal mol$^{-1}$ and diallyl-disulphide exhibited the least with binding energy value of -1.14 kcal mol$^{-1}$. As shown in Fig 2.5 (A), Alliin formed two bifurcated H-bonded interactions with three amino acids (arg154, thr179 and glu184) though carboxylate-O and amine-N atoms. In detail, O atom of carbonyl group (C=O) present in Alliin formed bifurcated H-bond interaction of length 2.54 Å and 2.74 Å with amine-N of Arg154 and carbonyl-O of Thr179 respectively. Similarly, amine-N of Alliin formed bifurcated H-bonding interaction of length 2.79 Å with carboxylate-O of Glu184 and 2.73 Å with carbonyl-O of Thr179. Notably, Allicin (Fig 2.5 (B)) and diallyl disulphide (Fig 2.5 (D)) did not participate in any H-bonded interactions while S-allyl cysteine (Fig 2.5 (C)) formed three H-bonding interaction with three amino acids. In detail, two oxygen atoms of carboxylate group present in S-allyl cysteine formed H-bond of lengths 2.76 Å and 2.78 Å with amine-N of Asn156 and amine-N of Gln155 respectively. In addition, amine-N of S-allyl cysteine formed H-bond of 2.52 Å with carbonyl-O of Glu153. From this observation, it can be concluded that diallyl disulphide and S-allyl cysteine shared similar active site amino acids like His 188, Ile 149, Ser 152 and Arg 154 whereas Alliin and Allicin have shown almost similar binding energies of -1.87 kcal mol$^{-1}$ and -1.86 kcal mol$^{-1}$ respectively.

Fig 2.5 Docking Poses of the Four Phytocompounds of Garlic with Proapoptotic Protein Bax

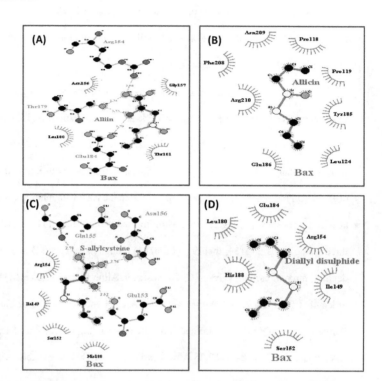

Ligplot representation of molecular docking analysis showing hydrogen bond interaction of Bax with Alliin(A), Allicin(B), S-allyl cysteine(C) and Diallyl disulphide(D).

Table 2.5 Binding Energy and Docking Site of Phytocompounds of Garlic (Alliin, Allicin, S-Allyl Cysteine and Diallyl Disulphide) with Bax

| S. No | Protein-Ligand Complex | Active Site (Amino Acids) | Hydrogen Bonds | Binding Energy (kcal mol$^{-1}$) |
|---|---|---|---|---|
| 1 | Bax-Alliin | Leu 180, Thr 181 | Arg 154, Thr 179, Glu 184 | -1.87 |
| 2 | Bax-Allicin | Val 121, Ala 124 | — | -1.86 |
| 3 | Bax-S-allyl cysteine | Ser 152, Arg 187, Arg 154 | Glu 153, Gln 155, Asn 156 | -1.94 |
| 4 | Bax-Diallyl disulphide | Ile 149, Arg 154, His 188 | — | -1.14 |

The phytocompounds in ginger exhibited weak interactions with Bax having very low binding energies (Table 2.6). A least interaction was observed with [10]-Gingerol with lowest binding energy value of -0.1 kcal mol$^{-1}$. [6]-Gingerol and Zingerone showed almost similar binding energies of -0.92 kcal mol$^{-1}$ and -0.94 kcal mol$^{-1}$ respectively. The docking poses of proapoptotic protein Bax with ligands [6]-Gingerol(A), [8]-Shogal(B), [10]-Gingerol(C) and Zingerone(D) are shown in Fig 2.6. As shown in (I), O2 atom of carbonyl group (C10=O2) present in [6]-Gingerol formed bifurcated H-bonding interactions of length 2.81 Å and 2.93 Å with imine-N and amine-N of Arg210 respectively whereas [10]-Gingerol did not form any sort of H-bonding interaction (Fig 2.6(C)). [8]-Shogal formed multiple H-bonding interactions with different amino acids (Glu184, Arg187, His188 and Asp150) (Fig 2.6(B)). In detail, carboxylate-O of [8]-Shogal formed three H-bond interactions of length 2.77 Å, 3.01 Å and 2.59 Å with amine-N of Arg187, amine-N of Arg187 and imidazole-N of His188 respectively. In addition, carbonyl-O of [8]-Shogal formed bifurcated H-bonds of length 3.04 Å and 2.56 Å with amine-N of Arg154 and carboxylate-O of Glu184. In addition to H-bonding interaction of [8]-Shogal, imidazole-N of His188 formed H-bonds with carboxylate-O of Asp150 of length 2.93 Å. Similarly, Zingerone also formed multiple H-bonds with different amino acids (Fig 2.6 (D)). In details, carbonyl-O of Zingerone formed bifurcated H-bonds of length 2.92 Å and 3.07 Å with amine-N of Gln155 and amine-N of Asn156 respectively. Additionally, methoxy-O and hydroxyl-O of Zingerone enables H-bond with carbonyl-O of Ser152 (length 2.59 Å) and amine-N of Ile149 (length 2.51 Å).

Like Bax, the interactions of different phytocompounds in garlic with anti-apoptotic molecule Bcl2 were studied. The docking scores of Bcl2 with different phytocompounds in garlic generated by autodock are shown in Table 2.7 and the corresponding docking poses are

**Fig 2.6 Docking Poses of the Four Phytocompounds of Ginger with Proapoptotic Protein Bax**

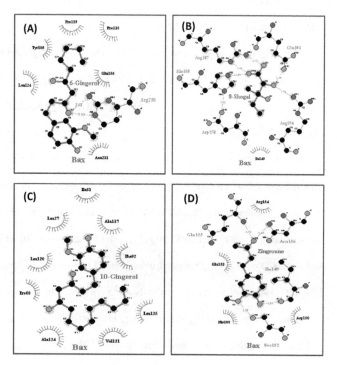

Ligplot representation of molecular docking analysis showing hydrogen bond interaction of Bax with [6]-Gingerol(A), [8]-Shogal(B), [10]-Gingerol(C) and Zingerone(D).

**Table 2.6 Binding Energy and Docking Site of Phytocompounds of Ginger ([6]-Gingerol, [8]-Shogal, [10]-Gingerol and Zingerone) with Bax**

| S. No | Protein-Ligand Complex | Active Site (Amino Acids) | Hydrogen Bonds | Binding Energy (kcal mol$^{-1}$) |
|---|---|---|---|---|
| 1 | Bax-[6]-Gingerol | Leu124, Pro119, Glu186 | Arg210 | -0.92 |
| 2 | Bax-[8]-Shogal | Ile149 | Asp150, Arg154, Glu184, His188, | -0.43 |
| 3 | Bax-[10]-Gingerol | Phe92, Leu120, Ala124, Leu125, | – | -0.1 |
| 4 | Bax-Zingerone | Glu153, Asp150, Arg154 | Ile149, Ser152, Gln155, Asn156 | -0.94 |

**Fig 2.7 Docking Poses of the Four Phytocompounds of Garlic with Anti-Apoptotic Protein Bcl2**

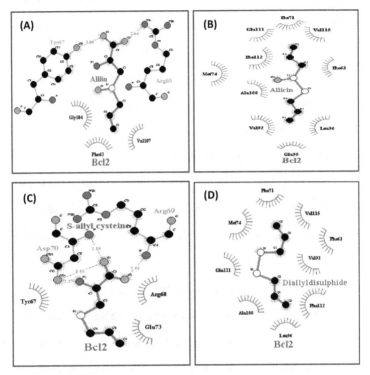

Ligplot representation of molecular docking analysis showing hydrogen bond interaction of Bcl2 with Alliin(A), Allicin(B), S-allyl cysteine(C) and Diallyl disulphide(D).

**Table 2.7 Binding Energy and Docking Site of Phytocompounds of Garlic (Alliin, Allicin, *S*-Allyl Cysteine and Diallyl Disulphide) with Bcl2**

| S. No | Protein-Ligand Complex | Active Site (Amino acids) | Hydrogen Bonds | Binding Energy (kcal mol$^{-1}$) |
|---|---|---|---|---|
| 1 | Bcl2-Alliin | Gly104, Phe63, Val107 | Arg66, Tyr67 | -3.36 |
| 2 | Bcl2-Allicin | Ala108, Val92, Phe112, Val 115 | – | -2.57 |
| 3 | Bcl2-*S*-allyl cysteine | Arg68, Tyr67 | Arg69, Asp70 | -3.11 |
| 4 | Bcl2-Diallyl disulphide | Phe112, Val92 | – | -2.65 |

shown in Fig 2.7. From the table, it was found that Alliin exhibited stronger interaction with Bcl2 than other phytocompounds with a relative higher binding energy of -3.36 kcal mol$^{-1}$. whereas Allicin exhibited a least weak interaction (-2.57 kcal mol$^{-1}$). From the docking poses analysis, it was found that the carboxylate group of Alliin formed two H-bonding interactions of length 3.0 Å and 2.64 Å with hydroxyl-O of Tyr67 and amine-N (NB1) of Arg66 respectively with a binding energy of -3.36 kcal mol$^{-1}$ (Fig 2.7 (A)). Allicin (Fig 2.7 (B)) and diallyl disulphide (Fig 2.7 (D)) did not participate in any H-bonding interactions whereas O1 atom of carboxylate group present in S-allyl cysteine (Fig 2.7 (C)) formed bifurcated H-bonds of length 2.85 Å and 3.05 Å with amine-N and carbonyl-O of Asp70 respectively. In addition, the other O2 atom of the carboxylic group present in S-allyl cysteine formed H-bond of length 2.86 Å with amine-N of Arg69.

Like garlic, interactions of Bcl2 with the four phytocompounds of ginger were explored. The docking scores by autodock analysis are outlined in Table 2.8 and the corresponding docking poses are shown in Fig 2.8. From the table, it was found that [8]-Shogal exhibited relatively higher interaction with Bcl2 with binding energy of -3.55 kcal mol$^{-1}$ while [10]-Gingerol showed the least interaction with a binding energy of -3.0 kcal mol$^{-1}$. As shown in Fig 2.8 (A), carbonyl group's O4 atom) and methoxy-O2 of [6]-Gingerol formed H-bonds of length 2.83 Å and 2.87 Å with carboxylate-O of Glu98 and amine-N of Asp107 respectively. The carboxylate-O3 of [8]-Shogal (Fig 2.8 (B)) formed two H-bonding interactions of length 2.69 Å and 2.95 Å with amine-N of Arg66 and hydroxyl-O of Try67 respectively however [10]-Gingerol did not participate in any H-bonding interactions (Fig 2.8 (C)). The methoxy-O of Zingerone formed H-bond of length 3.05 Å with carbonyl-O of Val92 (Fig 2.8 (D)).

**Fig 2.8 Docking Poses of the Four Phytocompounds of Ginger with Anti-Apoptotic Protein Bcl2**

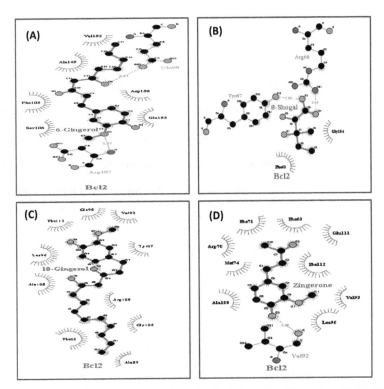

Ligplot representation of molecular docking analysis showing hydrogen bond interaction of Bcl2 with [6]-Gingerol(A), [8]-Shogal(B), [10]-Gingerol(C) and Zingerone(D).

**Table 2.8 Binding Energy and Docking Site of Phytocompounds of Ginger ([6]-Gingerol, [8]-Shogal, [10]-Gingerol and Zingerone) with Bcl2**

| S. No | Protein-Ligand Complex | Active Site (Amino Acids) | Hydrogen Bonds | Binding Energy (kcal mol$^{-1}$) |
|---|---|---|---|---|
| 1 | Bcl2-[6]-Gingerol | Phe105, Glu153, Ala149, Asp156 | Glu 98, Asp 107 | -3.45 |
| 2 | Bcl2-[8]-Shogal | Phe 63, Gly 104 | Arg 66, Tyr 67 | -3.55 |
| 3 | Bcl2-[10]-Gingerol | Ala108, Tyr67, Val92, Phe63, Gly104 | – | -3.0 |
| 4 | Bcl2-Zingerone | Leu96, Ala108, Phe112 | Val 92 | -3.23 |

In general, Bcl2 family proteins are considered as an evolutionarily conserved regulatory factor in apoptosis. Depending on the structure and function of Bcl2, they are divided into two groups such as antiapoptotic proteins and proapoptotic proteins. The former type (Group-I) includes Bcl-xL, Mcl-1 and Bcl-w proteins containing Bcl2 homology domains (BHI-4) whose primary function is the inhibition of pro-apoptotic proteins whereas the latter type (Group-II) contains Bad, Bax, Bak, BclxS, Bid Bik and Bim that stimulate apoptosis having only BH3 domains (Kam and Ferch 2000, Rastogi and Sinha 2010). From the above results, it can be concluded that [6]-Gingerol from ginger and Alliin from garlic might be used as potent Bcl2 inhibitors to suppress the malignancies of cancer.

## 2.4 Conclusion

In conclusion, among the different phytoconstituents present in ginger and garlic [6]-Gingerol in ginger and Alliin in garlic interact strongly with the pro-inflammatory markers (NFkB, COX-2) and Apoptotic markers (Bax and Bcl2). Accordingly [6]-Gingerol and Alliin were chosen for all molecular mechanistic studies in further *in vitro* experiments. However it doesnot mean that the other phytoconstituents donot exhibit possible activity. It helps us to identify the potential leads and narrow down the experimental studies.

# CHAPTER 3

## In-Vitro Studies on the Anticancer Potential of [6]-Gingerol and Alliin

# CHAPTER 3

## 3.1 Introduction

The aim of drug discovery is to develop protocols that engender unique and specific compounds that either inhibit or activate different processes in the cell and elicit therapeutic effects in humans. In this regard, basic science plays a central role in discovering new targets and physiological processes. The greatest advantage of *in vitro* assays however offer unique pathways for elucidating mechanisms of drug efficacy and demonstrating the biological process involved in the response to drugs. The development of *in vitro* assays is to tackle the demerits of *in vivo* assays upon screening various drugs and their efficiency and become a major research highlight of this arena. The *in vitro* assays could eventually produce trustworthy data for the early screening of drug molecules or compounds in the preclinical phase of drug development by replacing *in vivo* methods. As earlier as *in vitro* testing performed, one can save more time and cost associated with progressing unsuitable candidates through the pipeline by reducing the amount of animal testing and consequently reduce the overall cost of drug discovery (Li 2011). Various *in vitro* assays which are being developed for *in vitro* testing in drug development which include Chemical methods, Isolated organ bath studies and Cell culture based assays.

### 3.1.1 Chemical Methods

*In-vitro* assays are generally applied to evaluate the safety and efficiency of a drug in drug discovery and development. A classic example of screening candidate drug by chemical methods includes the antioxidant and free radical scavenging potential. Generation of reactive oxygen species, nitrogen species during a disease condition can be inhibited by the supplementation of anti-oxidants. Therefore, for reducing the risk of most diseases this has become an attractive therapeutic strategy. The rampant production of reactive oxygen species can be suppressed by free radical scavengers from natural origin and subsequently lipid peroxidation, DNA strand breaking and protein damage takes place which can provide protection to living organisms (Gill and Tuteja 2010). The major *in vitro* chemical assays employed so far for screening the antioxidant potential of drug molecules include *in-vitro* DPPH Radical Scavenging Activity, *in vitro* Lipid Peroxidation inhibition assay, *in- vitro* Nitric Oxide Scavenging Activity, Ferric reducing antioxidany potential (FRAP) assay, ORAC (oxygen radical absorbance capacity) and TEAC (Trolox equivalent antioxidant capacity) assays.

### 3.1.2 Isolated Organ Bath Studies

In drug discovery, isolated organ bath model is the classical pharmacological screening tool that offers biologically relevant structural and functional features. It supports both cell–cell and cell–extracellular matrix (ECM) interactions and defines both the efficacy and potency at a defined target, as well as the selectivity of a molecule. These are the crucial factor in the characterization of new therapeutic molecules. Traditionally, tissue-organ baths are used for the exploration of suggested tissue responses to pharmacological drug/agents (*in vitro* dose response experiments). This is also used to explore the physiology and pharmacology of tissue preparations from various species (chick, toad, rabbit, rat, guinea-pig, etc.) and generally are performed in a temperature controlled environment and perfused in oxygenated condition. This *in vitro* model retains closely the multi-cellular complexity, extra-cellular interactions, structural and functional features of the whole organ by mimicking biochemical capacity and the functional heterogeneity allowing the assessment of total metabolism and potential efficacy of a compound under conditions most like the *in vivo* situation. Although this model is independent of the systemic influences of *in vivo* preparations, due to its expensive setup, very short life span and different ethical issues this is not extensively used in drug toxicity assessment.

### 3.1.3 Cell Culture Assays

Cell culture based assays use cell lines which provide a homogenous population of cells and can be continuously sub-cultured through an acceptable number of passages to provide large numbers of cells in a short period of time. *In vitro* assays using cell line model systems can be applied to predict anticancer drug response and to understand the mechanisms of drug action (Voskoglou-Nomikos, Pater et al. 2003). Cell based assays use well-controlled systems and could be utilized to perform various high-throughput assays in a relatively short time period for any given drug or combinations of drugs with fewer confounding factors than *in vivo* assays. The various cell culture based assays used to check the anticancer effect of drug molecules include Cell viability assay, *In vitro* sulphorhodamine assay (SRB), Apoptosis detection by different staining procedures (AO/EB, DAPI, PI), Annexin V assay, Scratch assay etc.

Identifying the anticancer potential of specific drug molecules on different cancers can be tested on appropriate cell lines and it paves way to pin down specific targets. The present chapter outlines the studies involving *in vitro* assays used to identify the anticancer potential of ginger and garlic and its bioactive compounds.

### 3.2 Materials and Methods

### 3.2.1 Plant Material and Preparation of Aqueous Extract of Ginger and Garlic

From the local supermarket (originally from Pondicherry, India), both fresh ginger as well as fresh garlic were obtained. Before sample preparation, the ginger was washed thoroughly and sliced into small pieces. The dried powder samples were obtained after shade drying (37 °C) and grinding. Five hundred gram of ginger powder was collected and extracted with double distilled water by cold percolation. Likewise, fresh garlic were peeled of completely and cut in to small pieces before performing extraction. In a similar manner five hundred grams of dried garlic was weighed and ground into a coarse powder before extraction. The aqueous extracts were filtered and concentrated in a rotary evaporator at less than 40 °C under vacuum. Finally, the percentage yield of whole aqueous extract of fresh ginger, dried ginger, fresh garlic and dried garlic was calculated. Before quantification undissolved material was removed by centrifugation at 5000 $g$ for 10 minutes. The supernatant was then filtered through a 0.45 µm filter and stored in 4 °C for future use.

### 3.2.2 Quantification of Bioactive Lead Compounds in Ginger and Garlic

Based on the *in-silico* docking studies the identified active compounds [6]-Gingerol and Alliin were quantified in the fresh and dried ginger and garlic extracts by using HPLC.

**Preparation of Standards**

Standard solutions of known quantity of the [6]-Gingerol and Alliin (0.1 mg/mL) were prepared separately, dissolved in 99% ethanol in different concentrations.

**Preparation of Ginger and Garlic Extract**

Aqueous extract of ginger and garlic (10 mg/mL) were dissolved in ethanol and filtered twice through a Whatman filter paper: 1 and then with nitrocellulose membrane (2 µm).

**Chromatographic Conditions**

Quantification of [6]-Gingerol, the abundant phytoconstituent from both fresh and dried ginger was done by HPLC (Shimadzu LC solution). A known volume of aqueous extracts was prepared and an aliquot was then injected into C18 reverse phase HPLC column for the quantification of [6]-Gingerol. A mixture of MeOH/$H_2O$, 75:25 (v/v) as mobile phase A and a solution of acetonitrile/$H_2O$ 67:33 (v/v) as mobile phase B were used at a flow rate of 0.8

mL/minute. The UV detection was performed at 280 nm (Hiserodt, Franzblau et al. 1998, da Silva, Becceneri et al. 2012). Similarly, Alliin, the abundant phytoconstituent both from fresh and dried garlic was quantified by using a solution of 0.1% Trifluoroacetic acid (TFA) in $H_2O$ as mobile phase A and a solution of 0.1% Trifluoroacetic acid (TFA) in acetonitrile as mobile phase B at a flow rate of 0.8 mL/minute. The UV detection was performed at 210 nm (Dethier, Laloux et al. 2012, Lee, Gupta et al. 2013). The peak area of Alliin in both the extracts was matched with standard Alliin (Sigma) and the quantity of Alliin in both the fresh and dried garlic extracts was determined.

### 3.2.3 Antioxidant Capacity and Free Radical Scavenging Assay

For exploring antioxidant activity and free radical scavenging property of plant materials, several assays are reported. Among them, Lipid Peroxidation inhibition assay, Nitric oxide scavenging assay, DPPH scavenging assay and FRAP assay are the most reliable and reproducible methods. Ginger, garlic and its two active compounds were subjected to these assays in various concentrations.

**DPPH Radical Scavenging Assay**

**Reagents**

i. DPPH (150 µM) in ethanol

ii. Ethanol

**Procedure**

The DPPH assay was performed with 10 µL of each concentration of test samples diluted with 190 µL of DPPH solution. The mixture was incubated for 20 minutes at 37 °C. Controls were treated in the same way except with the addition of test drug. The decrease in absorbance at 517 nm refers to the quenching of DPPH free radicals and with respect to the controls, the percentage inhibition was calculated by the formula described below (Koleva, Van Beek et al. 2002).

## Lipid Peroxidation Assay

**Reagents**

i. Ice-cold potassium chloride (0.15 M)

ii. $Fe_2SO_4$ (25 µM)

iii. Ascorbate (100 µM)

iv. $KHPO_4$ (10 mM)

v. 5% TCA

vi. Thiobarbutyric acid (TBA) 0.375% in 0.5 N hydrochloric acid and slightly warmed for complete solubilisation.

vii. Sample preparation: Aqueous extracts of ginger and garlic with a concentration of 1000 µg/mL to 1.5 µg/mL were prepared with water and filtered through a Whatman filter paper: 1. [6]-Gingerol and Alliin with a concentration of 0.2-100 µM was prepared with ethanol.

**Procedure**

Lipid peroxidation was determined from the solution containing a mixture of 100 µL each of ferrous sulphate, ascorbate and potassium dihydrogen phosphate along with 10% of liver homogenate prepared in ice cold potassium chloride which was pre-incubated with various concentrations of test drugs. Finally, it was made up to 3 mL with distilled water and incubated for 1 h at 37 °C. Addition of 1 mL of 5% TCA and 1 mL of TBA was performed to arrest the reaction followed by boiling the tubes for 30 minutes in a boiling water bath maintained at 60 °C. Tubes were centrifuged at 3500 rpm for 10 minutes. Control tubes were treated in the same way except the addition of test drugs. Estimation of thiobarbituric acid reactive substances (TBARS) level was measured at an absorbance of 532 nm (Ohkawa, Ohishi et al. 1979). With respect to the controls, the percentage inhibition of lipid peroxidation was calculated.

**Ferric Reducing Antioxidant Power Assay**

**Reagents**

i. Acetate buffer (300 mM)

ii. 2,4,6-Tris(2-pyridyl)-s-triazine (TPTZ; 10 mM) in 40 mM HCl

iii. $FeCl_3 \cdot 6H_2O$ (20 mM)

iv. FRAP Reagent

Standard: 10:1:1 (Acetate buffer: TPTZ: $H_2O$)

Sample: 10:1:1 (Acetate buffer: TPTZ: $FeCl_3 \cdot 6H_2O$)

**Procedure**

The test system contained 40 µL sample mixture containing 0.2 mL of distilled water and 1.8 mL of FRAP reagent. After incubating the sample at 37 °C for 10 minutes, the absorbance of the reaction mixture was performed at 593 nm spectrophotometrically (Benzie and Strain 1996). As standard, 1 mmol/L $FeSO_4$ was used. The result was determined as FRAP value which implies the concentration of antioxidants (having a ferric reducing ability) to that of 1 mmol $FeSO_4$ per gram of sample.

### 3.2.4 *In-Vitro* Anti-inflammatory Potential by Cyclooxygenase (COX 2) Inhibitory Activity

Cyclooxygenase (COX-2) Inhibitory assay was undertaken to assess the probable mode of action of test drug. The inhibitory potential of [6]-Gingerol and Alliin were performed using the Cyclooxygenase Inhibitory Screening Assay kit (Catalogue no. 560131), Cayman Chemical, USA.

**Reagents**

i. Cyclooxygenase Inhibitory Screening Assay kit

ii. Preparation of test drugs: Both the test drugs were solubilized in methanol and made into concentration range of 0-500 µM.

**Procedure**

To perform this assay EIA buffer, Prostaglandin screening standards, Background samples, Cox II 100% initial activity samples, COX-2 inhibitor sample, prostaglandin screening ACHE tracers and antiserum were prepared according to the protocol mentioned in the catalogue. To the NSB wells, 100 µL EIA buffer was added and kept as duplicate wells. 50 µL EIA buffer was also added to B0 wells and kept duplicate. Standards of different concentrations of 50 µL were added to their respective wells. Thereafter 50 µL of COX-2 100% IA sample and COX-2 inhibitor sample were taken in their respective wells. Then 50 µL of tracer was added to all the wells except blank. 50 µL of antiserum was added to all the wells except blank and NSB wells to initiate the reaction followed by incubation of the 96 well plate in dark at room temperature for 18 h. After incubation, the plate was washed with wash buffer for five times. Then, 200 µL of chromogen was added to each well to initiate the reaction. The 96 well plate was covered and kept on a shaker for 55-90 minutes and finally the absorbance was taken at 420 nm using a ELISA plate reader. The percentage inhibition was calculated using the following formula:

$$\% \text{ Inhibition} = \frac{\text{OD of 100\% IA} - \text{OD of inhibitor sample} \times 100}{\text{OD of 100\% IA}}$$

### 3.2.5 Evaluation of Anticancer Potential

Cytotoxicity tests are imperative to rationalize the concentration range of bioactive leads providing significant data on parameters such as genotoxicity, induction of mutations or programmed cell death. By determining the half maximal inhibitory concentration dose at which 50% of the cells are affected (i.e. $TC_{50}/IC_{50}/EC_{50}$), the responses of single compounds in different systems or of several compounds in individual systems can be compared quantitatively. Cell viability assay (MTT) which identifies cell death and the $IC_{50}$ dose was performed to assess the antiproliferative property of the aqueous extracts of both Ginger (Fresh and Dried) and Garlic (Fresh and Dried) followed by their major phytoconstituents [6]-Gingerol and Alliin.

**Cell Culture and Growth Conditions**

AGS and INT-407 cell line was obtained from National Centre for Cell Sciences (NCCS, Pune) India. AGS is an adherent cell line derived from an adenocarcinoma of the stomach of a 54 year old Caucasian female with no prior anti-cancer treatment. Morphologically it is an epithelial cell which is hyper diploid in nature and has a doubling time of roughly 20 h. The mutant genes present in AGS cell lines are CDH1, CTNNB1, KRAS and PIK3CA. AGS cells could be useful for research related to stomach cancer of different forms. AGS cell line is a human gastric adenocarcinoma cell which was selected for the current study as it retains major functional characteristics of gastric cells (Barranco, Townsend et al. 1983). AGS cells on induction responds to external stimuli, henceforth the anticancer property of ginger, garlic and its active compounds were studied on this cell line. INT-407 (HeLa derivative) is an epithelial and adherent cell line from human cervix originally derived from the jejunum and ileum of a 2 month old Caucasian embryo and is used as a normal intestinal cell line against AGS cells

(Henle and Deinhardt 1957). The AGS cells and INT-407 cells were grown in T25 culture flasks containing Ham's F-12K (Kaighn's) medium along with 2 mM L-glutamine and 1500 mg/L sodium bicarbonate supplemented with 10% Fetal Bovine Serum (FBS), streptomycin (100 μg/mL) and penicillin (100 units/mL) which was maintained at 37 °C, in a humidified atmosphere containing 5% $CO_2$ / 95% air. Upon reaching 80% confluency, cells were detached using 0.2% Trypsin-EDTA solution.

### 3.2.5.1 Cell Viability Assay

**Reagents**

i. Dimethyl sulfoxide (DMSO)

ii. 3-(4, 5-dimethylthiazol-2-yl)-2,5-diphenyltetrazolium bromide (MTT): 5 mg/mL

iii. Phosphate buffered saline (PBS)

**Procedure**

The feasibility of AGS cells being treated with different amount of fresh ginger, dried ginger, [6]-Gingerol, fresh garlic, dried garlic extract and Alliin were assayed by the reduction of MTT to formazan insoluble dye (Mosmann 1983). To perform this, cells were plated into a 96-well plate ($1 \times 10^4$ cells per well in 200 μL of medium) and allowed to reach at confluent stage. Thereafter the cells were treated with different concentration of ginger and garlic extracts as well as with [6]-Gingerol and Alliin. After 24 h, cells were washed with PBS and incubated for 4 h at 37 °C with 50 μL of MTT (5 mg/mL). Finally, the removal of media took place followed by dissolving the formazan crystals in 200 μL of dimethyl sulfoxide (DMSO) and the absorbance was measured at 570 nm in a micro plate reader (Biorad imark) (Hansen, Nielsen et al. 1989).

### 3.2.5.2 Apoptosis Detection via Dual AO/EB Staining

**Reagents**

i. 10 mM Phosphate Buffered Saline, pH 7.4 (PBS)

ii. 100 µg/mL AO in PBS

iii. 100 µg/mL EB in PBS

**Procedure**

AO/EB dual staining was performed to differentiate between morphological features of apoptosis and necrosis (Cury-Boaventura, Pompéia et al. 2004). AGS cells were seeded in a six-well plate at a density of $1 \times 10^3$ cells per well and incubated overnight. Then various concentrations of [6]-Gingerol and Alliin was added and incubated for 24 h. The media was removed after incubation, and washed with PBS. From the mixture of Acridine Orange (AO; 100 µg/mL) and ethidium bromide (EBl; 100 µg/mL), 1 µL of dual fluorescent staining solution was taken and added to each suspension and a cover slip was used to cover the suspension. Using fluorescent microscope, the morphologies of stained cells was spotted (Nikon Eclipse T 100, Japan).

### 3.2.5.3 Wound Healing Assay

**Reagents**

i. 4% formalin

ii. Phosphate buffer saline

**Procedure**

Wound-healing assay was employed to monitor cell invasiveness as well as to determine the [6]-Gingerol and Alliin effects on cell migration. Mechanical wounds were introduced into confluent monolayers to determine whether the tested drugs could suppress the migration of

AGS cancer cells or not, and wound closure was measured by microscopy. The wound healing assays were conducted according to the methods described previously (Liang, Park et al. 2007). AGS cells were grown to 80-90% confluence in 6-well plates and then scratched to form a 100-mm "wound" using 200 µL sterile pipette tips. Detached cells were washed out using serum-free medium. The cells were then cultured for 24 h and 48 h in the presence or absence of [6]-Gingerol and Alliin in serum-free media and fixed with 4% formalin. 24 h and 48 h post-scratching, migration was documented and the images were recorded using a fluorescent microscope (Nikon Eclipse T 100, Japan). Periodically, the migration of treated cells into scratch was monitored by examining and imaging the culture plate.

### 3.2.5.4 Apoptosis Detection by Annexin-V Binding Assay

**Reagents**

i. DMSO (0.1-0.3%)

ii. Annexin-V binding buffer

iii. Annexin V conjugated with fluorescein isothiocyante (FITC)

iv. Propidium iodide (PI)

**Procedure**

To further confirm apoptosis, the percentage of cells that are actively undergoing apoptosis was determined by Annexin V-PE-based immunofluorescence. Labeling of cells with FITC-conjugated Annexin-V was performed according to the earlier method (Crowley, Marfell et al. 2016). Briefly, AGS cells were incubated for 30 minutes at 37 °C with 5 µL of 0.5 µg/mL FITC-conjugated Annexin-V in binding buffer and 5 µL of propidium iodide after 24 h of [6]-Gingerol and Alliin treatment by following the manufacturer protocol. Stained cells were washed two times in culture medium followed by the resuspension in PBS and finally analyzed by flow cytometer (Guava 8HT, Merck Millipore, Darmstadt, Germany). Distribution of cells in early and late phases of apoptosis was evaluated using Incyte software.

### 3.2.5.5 Flow Cytometric Analysis for Cell Cycle Distribution

**Reagents**

   i. Solution of propidium iodide

   ii. 0.1 % v/v of Triton X-100

   iii. 100 µg/mL of RNAase

**Procedure**

The most common method for assessing the cell cycle is to use flow cytometry to measure cellular DNA content. The hypodiploid DNA as well as cell cycle were determined similarly as earlier (Cao, Tang et al. 2015). Cells were plated in six well plate for 24 h with different doses of [6]-Gingerol and Alliin treatment. Thereafter, cells were washed twice with PBS and fixed with 70% ice cold ethanol overnight. Cells were then labeled with PI (0.05 mg/mL) in 1 mL of PBS containing 0.1% of Triton-X-100 and 50 µg of Ribonuclease for 30 minutes in dark at room temperature and analyzed for DNA content by using a Guava easy-cyte 8HT flow cytometer (Merck Millipore, Darmstadt, Germany) excited with blue laser (488 nm). Cells in different phases of the cell cycle were evaluated by the help of Incyte software.

### 3.2.5.6 Determination of Reactive Oxygen Species

**Reagents**

   i. 2,7-dichlorofluorescein diacetate (DCFDA)

   ii. Phosphate buffer saline

**Procedure**

Intracellular ROS was evaluated with DCFDA staining (Das, Suman et al. 2014) to identify the mode of action of the drugs. Cells were plated at a density of $2 \times 10^5$ cells mL$^{-1}$ in 6-well plates with different concentrations of [6]-Gingerol and Alliin treatment. After 24 h of treatment cells were washed with PBS and resuspended in 1 mL of complete media containing 10 µM DCFDA for 30 minutes. Finally, fluorescence was measured by a flow cytometer at an emission of 488 nm.

### 3.2.5.7 Measurement of Mitochondrial Membrane Potential

**Reagents**

i. Rhodamine 123

ii. Phosphate buffer saline

**Procedure**

Approximately $2 \times 10^5$ cells/well in a 12-well plate were treated with specified concentrations of [6]-Gingerol and Alliin, and incubated for specified time periods to identify the changes in the mitochondrial membrane potential ($\Delta\Psi_m$). Cells were harvested by centrifugation, washed twice in PBS, and then re-suspended in Rhodamine-123 (4 µM). The incubation was performed at 37 °C in dark for 30 minutes and the fluorescence intensity was measured in a flow cytometer previously described (Fulda and Kögel 2015).

### 3.2.5.8 Protein Extraction and Western Blot Analysis

**Reagents**

i. Cell lysis buffer

ii. Sodium dodecyl sulfate

iii. Running buffer

iv. Transfer buffer

**Procedure**

Immunoblot of apoptosis related proteins was done by a standard protocol (Bild, Yao et al. 2006). After treatment of AGS cells with respective concentrations of [6]-Gingerol and Alliin, cells were lysed with RIPA buffer (20 mM Tris-HCl, 1% SDS, pH 7.5, containing protease and phosphatase inhibitors) and centrifuged at 12000 g for 30 minutes. The collected supernatant was checked for total protein concentration by using the BCA protein assay kit (Pierce Biotechnology, Rockford, IL). For Western blotting equal amount of protein (50 µg) was resolved on a 12% SDS-polyacrylamide gel for electrophoresis and then transferred to PVDF membrane by a semidry transfer unit (Hoefer). Apoptotic proteins such as caspase 3, caspase 9, cytochrome c and Bax (Santa Cruz) and anti-apoptotic protein Bcl2 levels were detected and visualized on X-ray photographic film and quantified by Image J software by keeping β-Actin as a housekeeping gene.

### 3.2.6 Combination Study to Check Drug Interaction

The interaction or cooperation of two or more substances to produce a combined effect (greater, lesser or equal) than the sum of their separate effects is called as combination effect. Drug synergy occurs if it interacts in ways that enhance or magnify one or more additional effects. In most Indian culinary ginger garlic paste is used which mooted us to check the synergistic role of the active molecules in AGS cells. To evaluate the combination effects of [6]-Gingerol and Alliin as well as fresh aqueous extracts of ginger and garlic, cells were treated individually with serial dilutions of each drug and with both drugs simultaneously at a fixed ratio of doses that corresponded to the individual $IC_{50}$. Specifically, AGS gastric cancer cell line was exposed to various concentrations of Alliin and [6]-Gingerol at a ratio of 1:100. After

24 h of exposure, cell viability was measured using the MTT assay. In a similar manner, aqueous extract of both fresh ginger and fresh garlic were also studied for combination effect to check synergism. Chou and Talalay methods were used for the determination of drug interaction by combination index (Chou and Talalay 1984, Fujimoto-Ouchi, Sekiguchi et al. 2007). To determine the combination index, value, the analysis of the median effect was carried out using Compusyn software (Biosoft) wherein CI > 1: antagonistic effect, CI = 1: additive effect, CI < 1: synergistic effect.

### 3.2.7 Statistical Analysis

The results of the *In-vitro* studies were statistically evaluated and examined through one-way Analysis of Variance (ANOVA) using graph pad prism software (version 5.0) and Tukey's multiple comparison test and expressed as Mean ± SEM and a value of $p \leq 0.05$, $p \leq 0.01$ and $p \leq 0.001$ was considered significant.

### 3.3 Results and Discussion

### 3.3.1 Plant Material and Extract

The yield of whole aqueous extract of fresh ginger was found out to be 11.43% and yield of whole aqueous extract of dried ginger was found out to 6.58%. Likewise, the yield of whole aqueous extract of fresh garlic was found to 16.3% and the yield of whole aqueous extract of dried garlic was found to be 21.3%. The % yield of extract gives the % of phytoconstituents extracted out and was found comparable with the Ayurvedic Pharmacopeia monograph.

### 3.3.2 Chromatographic Analysis of Ginger and Garlic

The enormous rise in the global herbal drug and nutraceuticals market, the need for quality control, safety and efficacy data are required for international acceptance of drugs. Instrumental analytical methods like HPLC and HPTLC play a vital role in assessing the authenticity and quality of herbal drugs. In the present day, one of the most critical factors in developing pharmaceutical drug substances and drug products is to believe on HPLC analytical test methods ensuring meaningful data (Shabir 2003).

As per the HPLC analysis of both the form of garlic, fresh garlic contains highest content of Alliin (0.25 µg/mg) whereas dried garlic contains only (0.13 µg/mg) of Alliin. The Alliin content in fresh garlic is higher when compared to dried garlic. As it has been noted that garlic enzymatically produces Allicin when injured, but not all of the Alliin is being converted to Allicin (Prati, Henrique et al. 2014). A typical high-performance liquid chromatogram data of standard Alliin, fresh garlic, dried garlic extract is shown in Fig 3.1 (A, B, C) and Table 3.1. Similarly, in [6]-Gingerol the bioactive lead in ginger elutes immediately after the void volume, in retention time of 3.73. In the present study, the [6]-Gingerol content in the aqueous extract of fresh ginger is observed to be 6.11 µg/mg than the dried ginger extract which is found to be 0.407 µg/mg through the response of UV in the HPLC. Using HPLC, the results of this study, indicates that there is significant deviation in [6]-Gingerol concentration both in fresh and dried rhizomes. The concentration of [6]-Gingerol was observed more in fresh ginger than dried ginger Fig 3.2 (A, B, C) and Table 3.2. This is due to the fact that [6]-Gingerol undergoes dehydration reaction in dried ginger (Kou, Li et al. 2017).

### 3.3.3  *In-Vitro* Free Radical Scavenging Potential of Test Drugs

The antioxidant assays performed in this study measured the oxidative products at the early and final stages of oxidation. Antioxidants may act as free radical scavengers, reducing agents, chelating agents for transition metals, quenchers of singlet oxygen molecules and activators of antioxidative defense enzyme system to suppress the radical damages in biological systems (Venkatesh, Deecaraman et al. 2009, Murphy, Holmgren et al. 2011). Antioxidants

**Fig 3.1 Quantification of Alliin in Fresh and Dried Garlic Extracts**

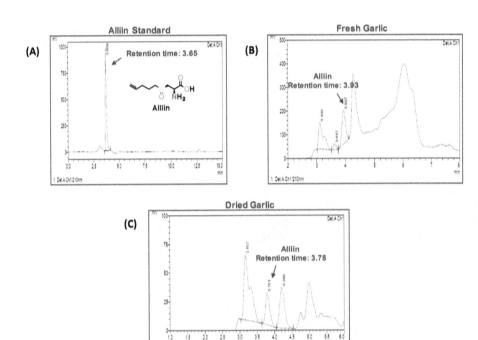

High-performance liquid chromatogram of standard Alliin (A), fresh garlic (B), dried garlic (C).

**Table 3.1 Quantification of Alliin from Garlic Extracts**

| Sample | Retention Time | Area | Height | Conc.(µg/mg) |
|---|---|---|---|---|
| Alliin | 3.65 | 1452268 | 100678 | 10.00 |
| Fresh Garlic | 3.93 | 179148 | 24743 | 0.25 |
| Dried Garlic | 3.78 | 231434 | 27639 | 0.13 |

**Fig 3.2 Quantification of [6]-Gingerol in Fresh and Dried Ginger Extracts**

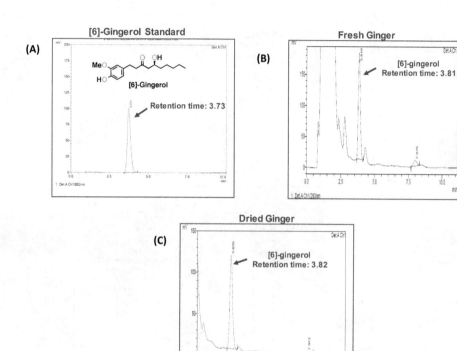

High-performance liquid chromatogram of standard [6]-Gingerol (A), fresh ginger (B), dried ginger (C).

**Table 3.2 Quantification of [6]-Gingerol from Ginger Extracts**

| Sample | Retention Time | Area | Height | Conc.(µg/mg) |
|---|---|---|---|---|
| [6]-Gingerol | 3.731 | 1452268 | 100678 | 5.000 |
| Fresh Ginger | 3.818 | 176622 | 170760 | 6.110 |
| Dried Ginger | 3.825 | 1189981 | 113445 | 0.407 |

thus seems to play an important role in the protection of human body against damage by reactive oxygen species (Ling, Tan et al. 2011, Peng, Hsu et al. 2011). Therefore, supplementation of antioxidants to inhibit the free radical-induced oxidative damage has become an attractive therapeutic strategy for reducing the risk of diseases. It has been proved that many plant species are serving as huge source of antioxidants and received therapeutic significance (Pari and Amudha 2011).

### 3.3.3(a) *In-Vitro* DPPH Radical Scavenging Activity

DPPH is a stable free radical but becomes a stable diamagnetic molecule upon accepting an electron or hydrogen radical. Therefore, in the presence of DPPH, antioxidants transfer an electron or hydrogen atom to it neutralizing its free radical character and convert it to 1,1-diphenyl-2-picryl hydrazine. The degree of discoloration from purple to yellow indicates the scavenging activity of the drug. The decrease in absorbance of DPPH radical is due to its reaction with antioxidant molecules and radical progress which results in the scavenging of the radical by hydrogen donation. Aqueous ginger and garlic extracts along with its active compounds, [6]-Gingerol and Alliin at various concentrations subjected to DPPH assay exhibited a dose dependent quenching of DPPH radicals. The results obtained are tabulated in Table 3.3(a). The *in vitro* results indicated that fresh ginger extract exhibited a significant free radical scavenging activity ($IC_{50}$ = 95.13 µg/mL) in comparison to dried ginger extract ($IC_{50}$ = 204.13 µg/mL). Likewise, fresh garlic extract showed an inhibition of 50.59 % at 64 µg/mL while dried garlic extract showed an inhibition of 50.07 % at 180 µg/mL. In comparison with standard antioxidant Ascorbic acid ($IC_{50}$ = 11 µM), [6]-Gingerol and Alliin exhibited DPPH scavenging potential with $IC_{50}$ of 34 µM and 30 µM respectively.

**Table 3.3(a) Anti-Oxidant Capacity of Test Drugs – Scavenging of DPPH**

| Dose (µM) | Ascorbic Acid | Dose (µM) | [6]-Gingerol | Alliin | Dose (µg/mL) | Fresh Ginger Extract | Dried Ginger Extract | Fresh Garlic Extract | Dried Garlic Extract |
|---|---|---|---|---|---|---|---|---|---|
| 0.2 | 20.16±1.6 | 0.2 | 4.16±1.6 | 2.16±1.4 | 1.5 | 1.2±0.1 | 0 | 1.12±0.2 | 0 |
| 0.4 | 28.67±1.6 | 0.4 | 8.67±1.8 | 7.67±1.6 | 3 | 4.94±0.5 | 3.94±0.4 | 5.94±0.8 | 3.94±0.3 |
| 0.6 | 35.73±1.3 | 0.6 | 15.73±1.9 | 13.73±1.3 | 7 | 8.33±1.3 | 7.33±1.4 | 9.33±1.4 | 6.33±1.2 |
| 0.8 | 40.05±1.1 | 0.8 | 24.05±2.5 | 24.05±2.1 | 15 | 12.76±1.5 | 14.76±1.6 | 12.76±1.4 | 13.76±1.4 |
| 1.0 | 42.65±2.1 | 1 | 32.65±2.9 | 31.65±2.8 | 30 | 23.60±1.9 | 18.60±1.3 | 27.60±2.0 | 19.60±1.8 |
| 20 | 60.79±4.1 | 20 | 43.65±3.2 | 42.65±3.1 | 62 | 45.08±3.4 | 25.08±2.4 | 48.08±3.6 | 26.08±1.9 |
| 40 | 65.88±1.4 | 40 | 61.79±3.9 | 62.79±3.8 | 125 | 73.98±3.6 | 32.98±2.9 | 62.98±3.2 | 31.98±2.6 |
| 60 | 68.25±2.6 | 60 | 69.25±3.6 | 66.25±3.6 | 250 | 85.85±4.2 | 78.85±4.3 | 75.85±4.1 | 68.85±3.2 |
| 80 | 70.82±2.9 | 80 | 72.82±3.9 | 71.82±3.8 | 500 | 90.99±4.8 | 80.99±4.6 | 82.99±4.4 | 70.99±3.6 |
| 100 | 75.25±2.8 | 100 | 75.25±3.92 | 80.25±4.2 | 1000 | 92.66±4.9 | 90.66±4.8 | 89.66±3.7 | 72.66±2.6 |

Results are expressed as % of free radical (DPPH) scavenged by the test drug, mean ± SEM.

### 3.3.3(b) *In-Vitro* Lipid Peroxidation Inhibition Assay

Thiobarbituric acid (TBA) test is one of the most commonly used assay for checking lipid peroxidation which involves the formation of malonaldehyde (MDA). TBA reacts with malonaldehyde, the byproduct of lipid peroxidation to form a pink chromogen, which is detected spectrophotometrically at 530 nm. Effect of ginger and garlic along with its active compounds, [6]-Gingerol and Alliin on the formation of lipid peroxides estimated in terms of thiobarbituric acid reactive substances (TBARS) production from thiobarbituric acid (TBA) is shown in Table 3.3(b). In the present study, lipid peroxide generation by $Fe^{2+}$-ascorbate in rat liver homogenate seems to be suppressed by fresh ginger extract with an $IC_{50}$ value of 95.23 µg/mL. Fresh ginger extract shows significant lipid peroxidation inhibition activity when compared to dried ginger extract which showed poor activity with an $IC_{50}$ = 308.47 µg/mL which reflects their less efficiency to suppress the generation of lipid peroxides. In a similar manner, fresh garlic extract showed to have a better $IC_{50}$ value of 86.23 µg/mL in comparison to dried garlic extract ($IC_{50}$ = 208.47 µg/mL).

In the case of pure compounds, [6]-Gingerol was found to show an $IC_{50}$ value of 54 µM while Alliin showed an $IC_{50}$ value of 48 µM which are comparable with proven antioxidant standard Ascorbic acid ($IC_{50}$ = 41 µM).

### 3.3.3(c) Ferric Reducing Antioxidant Power Assay

FRAP assay is considered as a novel method for assessing "antioxidant power" where reduction of ferric ion to ferrous ion at low pH causes a colored ferrous-tripyridyl triazine complex which can be monitored at 593 nm. The absorption readings are related to the reducing power of the electron donating antioxidants present in the test compound (Benzie and Strain 1996). In the present study, the pure compounds [6]-Gingerol showed a FRAP value as 45.0 ±

**Table 3.3(b) Anti-Oxidant Capacity of Test Drugs – Inhibition of Lipid Peroxidation**

| Dose (µM) | Ascorbic Acid | [6]-Gingerol | Alliin | Dose (µg/mL) | Fresh Ginger Extract | Dried Ginger Extract | Fresh Garlic Extract | Dried Garlic Extract |
|---|---|---|---|---|---|---|---|---|
| 0.2 | 07.88±1.9 | 5.14±0.8 | 4.14±0.8 | 1.5 | 1.3±1.0 | 1.12±0.2 | 1.4±0.3 | 3.14±0.8 |
| 0.4 | 13.34±3.2 | 5.68±0.8 | 8.68±0.9 | 3 | 6.82±1.2 | 2.02±2.1 | 5.82±1.2 | 7.20±1.4 |
| 0.6 | 24.54±1.6 | 14.31±1.3 | 16.31±1.5 | 7 | 12.92±2.4 | 6.12±2.3 | 12.82±1.5 | 10.67±1.5 |
| 0.8 | 29.57±1.4 | 14.90±1.4 | 18.90±1.7 | 15 | 26.12±2.3 | 9.89±2.4 | 17.92±1.6 | 16.58±1.7 |
| 1.0 | 34.14±2.6 | 16.67±1.5 | 26.67±2.1 | 30 | 35.89±2.7 | 11.01±2.5 | 25.12±2.3 | 22.13±1.9 |
| 20 | 41.57±4.9 | 23.60±1.7 | 33.60±2.3 | 62 | 41.01±3.1 | 13.20±2.5 | 33.60±2.5 | 36.60±2.3 |
| 40 | 48.08±2.4 | 31.98±2.4 | 41.57±2.9 | 125 | 59.25±3.6 | 19.66±2.6 | 69.25±3.6 | 42.57±2.9 |
| 60 | 61.52±2.0 | 61.79±3.1 | 59.25±3.2 | 250 | 61.79±4.1 | 33.60±2.7 | 74.85±3.2 | 55.92±3.5 |
| 80 | 64.64±2.3 | 69.25±3.6 | 62.98±3.4 | 500 | 67.25±4.6 | 65.98±3.6 | 80.99±4.8 | 63.25±3.6 |
| 100 | 71.82±2.9 | 75.82±3.9 | 68.98±3.6 | 1000 | 72.82±4.9 | 69.98±3.6 | 90.66±4.9 | 65.25±3.8 |

Results are expressed as % of free radicals scavenged by the test drugs, mean± SEM.

Table 3.3(c) Anti-Oxidant Capacity of Test Drugs – Ferric Reducing Antioxidant Power (FRAP)

| Dose (µM) | Ascorbic Acid | Dose (µM) | [6]-Gingerol | Alliin | Dose (µg/mL) | Fresh Ginger Extract | Dried Ginger Extract | Fresh Garlic Extract | Dried Garlic Extract |
|---|---|---|---|---|---|---|---|---|---|
| 0.2 | 0 | 0.2 | 1.1±1.6 | 0 | 1.5 | 1.4±0.5 | 1.5±0.4 | 1.3±0.6 | 0 |
| 0.4 | 10.1±1.6 | 0.4 | 10.4±1.5 | 11.1±1.5 | 3 | 11.6±1.7 | 10.6±1.3 | 2.4±1.5 | 1.4±1.2 |
| 0.6 | 12.4±2.3 | 0.6 | 10.6±1.7 | 14.4±1.6 | 7 | 12.0±1.8 | 12.1±1.4 | 10.6±1.7 | 5.6±1.3 |
| 0.8 | 15.6±2.3 | 0.8 | 12.0±1.8 | 18.6±1.7 | 15 | 15.4±1.8 | 12.4±1.8 | 32.0±2.3 | 12.0±1.4 |
| 1.0 | 23.0±2.2 | 1 | 20.4±2.6 | 20.0±1.9 | 30 | 16.5±1.9 | 22.8±2.4 | 43.6±2.4 | 22.6±1.5 |
| 20 | 25.4±2.3 | 20 | 22.5±1.9 | 24.1±2.7 | 62 | 18.4±2.4 | 30.7±1.9 | 47.3±2.6 | 23.8±1.7 |
| 40 | 28.9±2.4 | 40 | 32.7±2.6 | 26.17±2.7 | 125 | 22.46±2.5 | 33.73±2.4 | 55.45±2.9 | 30.8±2.3 |
| 60 | 38.4±2.3 | 60 | 45.0±2.5 | 39.19±2.7 | 250 | 34.5±2.8 | 35.8±2.3 | 58.47±2.6 | 43.86±2.6 |
| 80 | 42.5±2.2 | 80 | 39.04±2.6 | 32.2±1.7 | 500 | 43.96±3.5 | 36.4±2.5 | 63.5±3.6 | 45.9±2.7 |
| 100 | 44.6±2.6 | 100 | 38.1±2.62 | 32.5±1.9 | 1000 | 43.5±3.4 | 34.6±2.4 | 63.2±3.6 | 53.94±3.5 |

The antioxidant capacity based on the ability to reduce ferric ions of sample was calculated from the linear calibration curve and the FRAP values are expressed as mmol of $Fe^{2+}$/g sample.

2.5 equivalent mmol of $Fe^{2+}$/g sample in 80 µM concentration whereas alliin has higher FRAP value of 39.19 ± 2.7 at 60 µM concentration than standard Ascorbic acid (44.6 ± 2.6) at 100 µM. The four extracts tested fresh ginger extract, dried ginger extract, fresh garlic extract and dried garlic extract showed FRAP value of 43.96 ± 2.5, 36.4 ± 1.5, 63.5 ± 3.6 and 53.94 ± 2.5 equivalent mmol of $Fe^{2+}$/g samples, respectively. The results are tabulated in Table 3.3(c).

### 3.3.4 *In-Vitro* Anti-Inflammatory Potential

The antioxidant and anti-inflammatory potential displayed by phytocompounds contribute significantly to the oxidative stress related disorders like diabetes and cancer. [6]-Gingerol and Alliin has shown a better antioxidant potential in the previous result. Hence, to estimate the anti-inflammatory potential of the above two bioactive leads, COX-2 inhibitory assay was performed.

COX-2 is a bifunctional enzyme which is responsible for the biosynthesis of prostaglandins under acute and chronic conditions and possess both cyclooxygenase and peroxidase activities (Hinz and Brune 2002). Normal tissues express low levels of COX-2 but in inflammation and injury, COX-2 has known to express in high levels by the pro-inflammatory mediators and inhibition of COX-2 mainly accounts for the anti-inflammatory effect of drugs. Hence, COX-2 is regarded to be the target for the anti-inflammatory activity of non-steroidal drugs. Compounds which can specifically inhibit COX-2 without any side effect might have potent therapeutic actions like nonsteroidal anti-inflammatory drugs (NSAIDS). The present study reveals the anti-inflammatory potential of [6]-Gingerol and Alliin at various concentrations ranging from 0-500 µg/mL which was compared with a standard COX inhibitor Diclofenac (Fig 3.3). [6]-Gingerol showed a maximum percentage of inhibition of 52.0 % at 250 µg/ml with an $IC_{50}$ value of 230 µg/mL and Alliin showed a maximum percentage of

**Fig 3.3 COX-2 Inhibitory Assay of [6]-Gingerol and Alliin with Diclofenac**

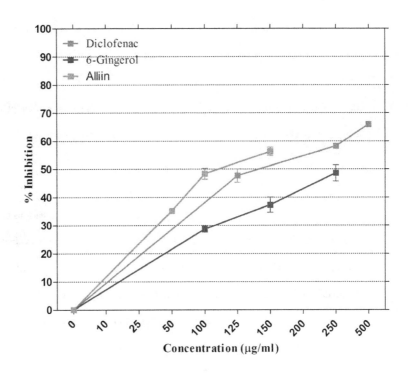

Values are expressed in Mean ± SEM in triplicates for each group in different concentrations

inhibition of 58% at 150 µg/ml with an $IC_{50}$ value of 145.70 µg/ml whereas Diclofenac showed a maximum percentage inhibition of 68% at 500 µg/ml with an $IC_{50}$ value of 490.5 µg/ml. Hence, this study displayed a potent anti-inflammatory potential of Alliin which is greater than [6]-Gingerol and which can be used as a potent COX-2 inhibitor in comparison to Diclofenac.

### 3.3.5 Cell Viability Potential-MTT Assay

MTT cell viability assay is a method widely recommended for examining the cytotoxic effect of xenobiotics, assessing proliferation rates, and analyzing cell activity by the reduction of MTT by viable cells in culture (Abid, Rouis et al. 2012). MTT assay was used to evaluate the reduction of viability of cell cultures in the presence and absence of the plant drug. Hence, cell viability assay was performed for [6]-Gingerol and Alliin (5 µM, 10 µM, 30 µM, 50 µM, 100 µM), 150 µM, 200 µM, 250 µM and 300 µM) in both AGS and INT-407 cell line while the extracts of ginger and garlic (1.5 µg/mL, 3 µg/mL, 7 µg/mL, 15 µg/mL, 30 µg/mL, 62 µg/mL, 125 µg/mL, 250 µg/mL, 500 µg/mL, and 1000 µg/mL) were tested in various concentrations in AGS cell line. Results obtained in Fig 3.4(A)-(C) show the cell viability evaluated after 24 h of incubation with [6]-Gingerol and Alliin and the extracts of ginger and garlic. [6]-Gingerol is found to inhibit cell growth till a concentration of about 300 µM, beyond which showed reduced cell viability when compared to the control. Like [6]-Gingerol, Alliin also was found to be non-toxic till 50 µM and showed only 50% viability at a higher concentration of 100 µM. In the case of normal intestinal cell INT-407, neither Alliin nor [6]-Gingerol induced proliferation or inhibited the cell growth. The extracts of ginger and garlic was also shown to be toxic over a range of concentration (300 µg/mL-1000 µg/mL). Based on the cell viability results, the efficacy studies were performed till a concentration of 100 µM ($IC_{50}$) value for Alliin and till a concentration of 250 µM ($IC_{50}$) value for [6]-Gingerol. To pin down and to explicate the

**Fig 3.4 Cytotoxic Effect of Test Drugs on AGS Cells**

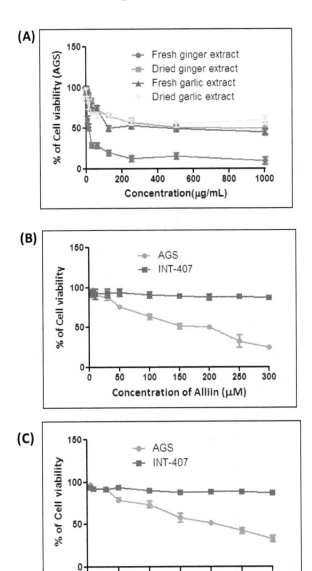

MTT cell viability assay for Ginger, Garlic extract on AGS cells (A), [6]-Gingerol in AGS and INT-407 cells (B) Alliin in AGS and INT-407 cells (C). The cell viability profiles were determined from triplicates of three independent experiments using the MTT assay after 24h exposure of cells to test compounds. Results are expressed in Mean ± SEM

mechanistic study of the more potent compounds, the above two mentioned compounds were subjected to different apoptosis assays.

### 3.3.6 Apoptosis Detection by AO/EB Staining

AO/EB Staining can identify some of the distinctive morphological features of apoptosis. A marked change in the morphology of AGS cells were observed which were characterized by round and floating cells gradually increasing from concentrations 50-100 μM in Alliin and from 100-250 μM in the case of [6]-Gingerol within 24 h of treatment. AGS cells treated with [6]-Gingerol and Alliin stained by acridine orange/ethidium bromide (AO/EB) dual stain evaluate the nuclear morphology of apoptotic cells. Cells stained green represent viable cells, whereas yellow staining represented early apoptotic cells, and reddish or orange staining represents late apoptotic cells (Liu, Liu et al. 2015). In control cell, substantial apoptosis was not identified which is represented by green colour live cells comprising normal and large nucleus. The apoptotic cells in their early stages, exhibited hemispherical shaped nuclei stained with AO which was detected in the experimental group (100 μM) of [6]-Gingerol and (50 μM) Alliin. However, proliferation of early stage apoptotic cells was observed with rising the concentration of (250 μM) [6]-Gingerol and (100 μM) of Alliin. The apoptotic potential of [6]-Gingerol and Alliin on the AGS cells was confirmed because late stage apoptotic cells that are concentrated and asymmetrical localized orange nucleus stained with EB was seen in both low and high concentrations (Fig 3.5 (A) and (B)). So, it confirms that [6]-Gingerol and Alliin significantly induced apoptosis in gastric cancer cells. It is interesting to note that [6]-Gingerol and Alliin treated cells showed significant morphological changes like cell shrinkage and reduced cell density with respect to untreated cells. Similar result was also observed by [6]-Shogal, one of the bioactive compound from ginger which induces apoptosis in human

**Fig 3.5 Morphological Features of Apoptosis in AGS Cells Detected by AO/EB Staining**

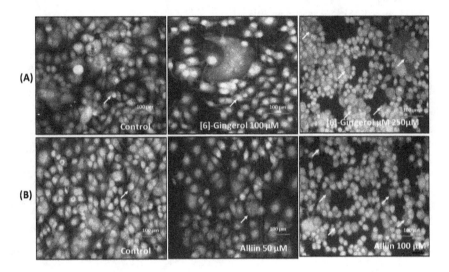

Acridine orange/Ethidium bromide dual staining of AGS cells by the treatment of [6]-Gingerol (A) and Alliin (B) in various concentrations in comparison control cells. The arrows in control cells show the appearance of normal healthy cells whereas the indicated arrows in treated cells confirm the presence of early (yellow-green) and late apoptotic cells (orange).

colorectal carcinoma (COLO 205) cells (Pan, Hsieh et al. 2008). Similarly allicin, one of the bioactive lead from garlic has shown antiproliferative activity in gastric cancer (SGC-7901) cells (Shao, Zhang et al. 2012).

### 3.3.7 *In-Vitro* Scratch Assay

The *in-vitro* scratch assay is the most suitable method to study the regulation of cell migration in relation to extracellular matrix (ECM) and cell–cell interactions (Liang, Park et al. 2007). This assay is one of the simplest and economical method. Scratch assay was done to judge the effects of [6]-Gingerol and Alliin on AGS cell migration. In the present study, a significant proportion of control AGS cells had migrated to the wound created after 24 h and 48 h. Conversely, cell migration was not observed in cells treated with [6]-Gingerol and Alliin (Fig 3.6(A) and (B)). The two compounds at inhibitory dose concentration of 50 for 24 h and 48 h inhibited cellular migration to the scratched zone. However, in control cells, the movement of cells was time dependent and hence cells moved slowly and were able to close the patch after 24 h. Notably, in case of cells treated with [6]-Gingerol and Alliin, such movement of cells was not observed. Additionally, due to the round shape of treated cells, they were weakly bound with the substratum when compared to control cells. The effect of [6]-Gingerol on inhibition of cell migration in MDA-MB-231 cells were well explored in some earlier studies (Lee, Seo et al. 2008). Saponins derived from some different Allium species reported to inhibit cell migration in B16 melanoma and 4T1 breast carcinoma cells (Yu, Zhang et al. 2015) while Allicin, one of the major organosulphur compound of garlic resulted in a significant decrease in the migration ratio in MCF-7 cells (Lee, Lee et al. 2015). Also a recent report found out that Diallyl trisulphide (DATS) one of active components in garlic oil inhibits the cell migration in A375 melanoma cells (Wang, Chu et al. 2017). From this assay, it was revealed

**Fig 3.6(A) Effect of [6]-Gingerol on Cellular Migration-Scratch Assay**

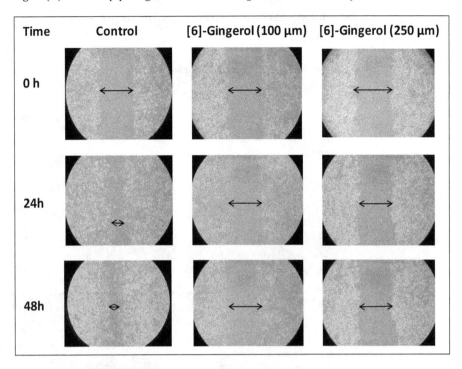

Cellular Migration-Scratch assay: the patches are created by scratching the monolayer. A significant reduction of cell migration reveals in presence of [6]-Gingerol (100 μM and 250 μM) for a time of 24h and 48h. The patch is completely covered within 24 h by the untreated cells, while limited area was covered in treated groups by fragmented way.

**Fig 3.6(B) Effect of Alliin on Cellular Migration-Scratch Assay**

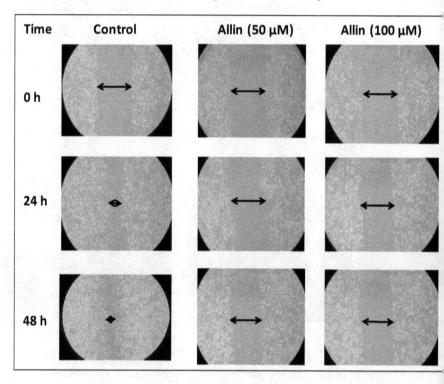

Cellular Migration-Scratch Assay: the patches are created by scratching the monolayer. A significant reduction of cell migration reveals in presence of Alliin (50μM and 100 μM) for a rime period of 24 h and 48 h. The patch is completely covered within 24 h by the untreated cells, while limited area was covered in treated groups by fragmented way.

that [6]-Gingerol as well as Alliin inhibit the cell migration in a dose and time dependent manner which might be one of the potent antimetastasis ability of both phytocompounds.

### 3.3.8 Quantitative Analysis of Apoptotic Cells by Annexin V/PI Staining

By taking into account the growth-inhibitory effects of the two compounds [6]-Gingerol and Alliin which were associated with the induction of apoptotic cell death, FITC-conjugated annexin V and PI double staining (detected by flow cytometry) was used as a measure to distinguish apoptotic cells (Gudarzi, Salimi et al. 2015, Hamzeloo-Moghadam, Aghaei et al. 2015). Annexin-V/PI staining was carried out by flow cytometry to check the effect of [6]-Gingerol as well as Alliin on the membrane flip-flop and externalization of phosphotedylserine. The combination of Annexin V-FITC and propidium iodide allows the differentiation among early apoptotic cells (annexin V-FITC-positive, PI-negative cells), late apoptotic cells (annexin V-FITC-positive, PI-positive cells) and necrotic cells (annexin V negative, PI positive). For both annexin V-FITC and PI, control cells were negative. Notably in Alliin treated cells the percentage of apoptotic cells increased from 0.01% in control cells to 56% whereas there is an increase in the percentage of apoptotic cells from 0.01% to 34.7% in [6]-Gingerol treated cells (Fig 3.7). Allicin, an organosulphur moiety from garlic was confirmed to increase the percentage of apoptotic cells in MDA-MB-231 than MCF7 breast cancer cells (Kim, Cho et al. 2016) and also in U251 glioma cells in a dose and time-dependent manner (Li, Jing et al. 2018). Similar results were also obtained in the case of [6]-Gingerol treated SW-480 colon cancer cells where the [6]-Gingerol concentration was 200 μM (Radhakrishnan, Bava et al. 2014). In another study, [10]-Gingerol in ginger significantly increased the percentage of apoptotic cells from 17.9% (control) to 85.7% (50 μM treated) in HCT116 human colon cancer cells (Ryu and Chung 2015). Therefore, the results of dual-colour flow cytometry analysis in the present

## Fig 3.7 Annexin V-FITC Assay for Detection of Apoptosis by Flow Cytometry

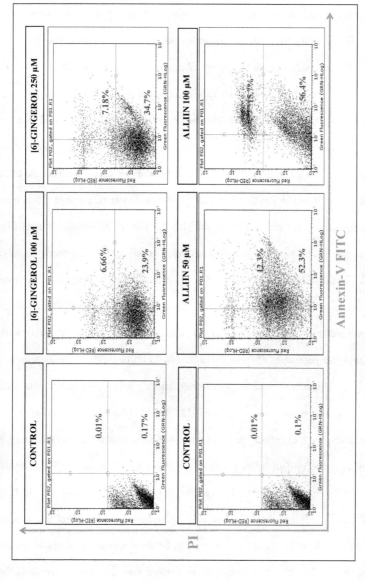

Representative analysis of apoptotic cell population in AGS cells after [6]-Gingerol and Alliin treatment. The results shown represent the mean± SEM of three independent experiments.

context confirmed that [6]-Gingerol as well as Alliin can induce apoptosis in AGS cells in a dose dependent manner.

### 3.3.9 Flow Cytometric Analysis of Apoptosis and Cell Cycle Arrest

In general cellular proliferation is predominantly linked to cell cycle progression (Kastan and Bartek 2004). To determine whether suppression of cell proliferation by [6]-Gingerol and Alliin results from inhibition of cell cycle progression, cell cycle analysis was carried out to evaluate the distribution of actively dividing cells before the induction of apoptosis. A large proportion of the cells accumulated in the G2/M phase at 24 h after the addition of 250 µM of [6]-Gingerol, indicates a growth arrest at the S/G2 phase transition (Fig 3.8(A)). Similar results were also observed in the case of cervical cancer (HeLa and CaSki) cells at 50 µM of [6]-Gingerol (Rastogi, Duggal et al. 2015). The results shown in Fig 3.8(B) represented that Alliin dose dependently increased the S phase population in AGS cells and a corresponding decrease of cells in G2/M phase which results in a growth arrest of S phase. Allicin, the active compound formed from Alliin in garlic cloves at a concentration of 30µM resulted in an increase in the percentage of cells in the G0/G1 and G2/M phases and a concomitant reduction in the S fraction in MCF-7 cells breast cancer cells (Hirsch, Danilenko et al. 2000). Allicin also increased the sub-G1 cell populations in MDA-MB-231 cells (Kim, Cho et al. 2016). Evidence revealed that various cell cycle regulators like cyclins, and their catalytic partner, Cdks noticeably control the cell cycle progression (Gallorini, Cataldi et al. 2012). In our study, the G2/M phase arrest in [6]-Gingerol treated cells might be due to the decrease in the levels of cyclin D1, cyclin E, and Cdk1 proteins in AGS cells whereas the S phase arrest of Alliin treated cells might be because of Cdk2 and Cdk4 proteins in AGS cells.

**Fig 3.8 Effect of [6]-Gingerol and Alliin on Cell Cycle Arrest in AGS Cells**

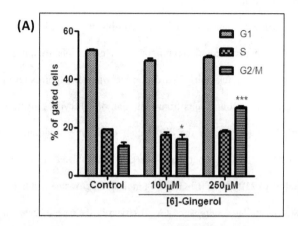

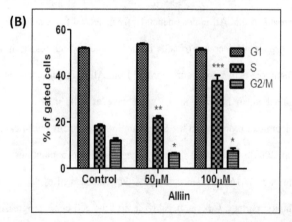

AGS cells were treated with [6]-Gingerol (A) and Alliin (B) respectively with the indicated concentrations for 24 h. Bars represent the percentage of gated cells present in each of the cell cycle stages: G1, S, G2/M or those that had apoptosed (n=3, * $p \leq 0.05$, ** $p \leq 0.01$, *** $p \leq 0.001$).

### 3.3.10 Measurement of Intracellular Reactive Oxygen Species

The cellular ROS generation is the outcome of the electron and proton transport through the inner membrane of mitochondria and mitochondria-mediated abnormal ROS is widely recognized as an aggravating factor in numerous human diseases (Valko, Leibfritz et al. 2007). ROS are believed to involve in several cellular functions, such as cell proliferation, differentiation, and apoptosis and have been proved to play a key role in cancer chemotherapy (Liou and Storz 2010). Increase in ROS level generation leads to potentially cytotoxic oxidative stress which are identified as apoptosis inducers and modulators (Trachootham, Lu et al. 2008). Many natural chemotherapeutic agents induce cytotoxicity which is mediated by the production of ROS. In this study, the intracellular ROS level in AGS cells treated with different concentration of [6]-Gingerol (100 µM and 250 µM) and Alliin (50 µM and 100 µM) was significantly elevated as compared with the control group cells. It is illustrated in Fig 3.9 (A) and (B) that [6]-Gingerol and Alliin triggered apoptosis associated with excessive ROS generation in AGS cells, demonstrating that both the compounds might exhibit anticancer activity by excessive generation of ROS. In an earlier study, 50 µM [6]-Gingerol induced a dose dependent increase in ROS generation in both K562 and U937 cells (Rastogi, Gara et al. 2014). Another study reported that intracellular ROS levels were also increased significantly in [6]-Gingerol treated human epidermoid carcinoma (A 431) cells in a dose dependent way (Nigam, Bhui et al. 2009). DATS, one of the principal constituents of garlic oil was shown to raise intracellular ROS generation in AGS cells (Choi 2017). Typically, AGS cells treated with [6]-Gingerol and Alliin recorded elevated ROS levels over vehicle treated control cells. It is worth mentioning that these compounds might act as potential modulators of apoptosis and prove to

**Fig 3.9 Detection of Reactive Oxygen Species (ROS) Generation**

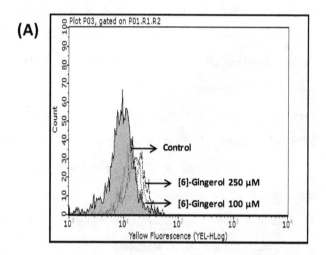

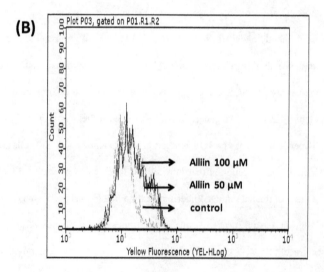

Effects of [6]-Gingerol (A) and Allin (B) on reactive oxygen species (ROS) generation in AGS cell line. Results (mean ± SEM) were calculated as percent of corresponding control values. The YEL-HLog on the X-axis denotes Reactive oxygen species generation and Cell count on the Y-axis.

be potent agents in mitigating the oxidative stress involved in cancerous lesions more specifically in gastric adenocarcinoma as evidenced by present study.

### 3.3.11 Measurement of Mitochondrial Membrane Potential

Mitochondria which is considered the powerhouse of cell also plays an important role in apoptosis. Various cellular stimuli cause irreversible apoptotic cell death by disrupting mitochondria. Thus the major parameter of mitochondrial function, $\Delta\Psi_m$ is acknowledged as an indicator of programmed cell death (Wang 2001). Many apoptotic signals transduce their death-inducing message through mitochondria. Depletion of the mitochondrial membrane potential $\Delta\Psi_m$ is an early marker of the apoptotic process (Hamzeloo-Moghadam, Aghaei et al. 2015). Due to increased metabolism, cancer cells exhibit increased $\Delta\Psi_m$ and test compounds that scrupulously promote mitochondrial membrane permeabilization are interesting drug candidates for drug development (Chen 1988, Fulda, Galluzzi et al. 2010). Treatment of AGS cells to various concentrations of [6]-Gingerol (100 µM and 250 µM) and Alliin (50 µM and 100 µM) for 24 h led to a noticeable loss of the mitochondrial membrane potential in a concentration as well as time dependent manner in comparison to control cells (Fig 3.10 (A) and (B)). Depolarization of $\Delta\Psi_m$ results in the loss of Rhodamine-123 from the mitochondria and a decrease in intracellular fluorescence along with the depletion of mitochondrial membrane potential ($\Delta\Psi_m$) in a dose-dependent manner in AGS cells. These results suggest that induction of apoptosis by [6]-Gingerol as well as Alliin may be due to the disruption of mitochondrial-related mechanisms. Quantitative data acquired by flow cytometer in the present study also supports the mitochondrial membrane potential depolarization convincingly where it decreased subsequently within a period of 24 h providing evidence of mitochondria mediated apoptosis. It is interesting to note that our study corroborates to earlier studies on different cell lines

**Fig 3.10 Measurement of Mitochondrial Membrane Potential (MMP)**

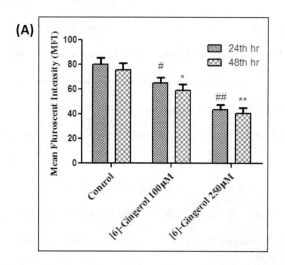

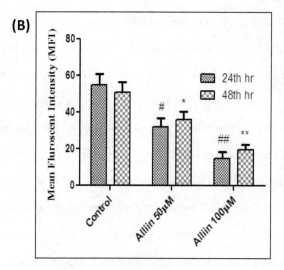

AGS cells were treated with [6]-Gingerol (A) and Alliin (B) at indicated concentrations over different time periods. ΔΨm was observed in a concentration as well as time dependent manner. Data represent the average values from triplicates of three independent experiments. #$P \leq 0.05$; ##$P \leq 0.01$ in comparison to control for 24th hr and *$P \leq 0.05$; **$P \leq 0.01$ in comparison to control for 48th h is considered significant.

wherein, [6]-Gingerol also displayed the depolarization of mitochondrial membrane potential in HeLa cells (Chakraborty, Bishayee et al. 2012) while in A431 cells, [6]-Gingerol treatment resulted in a dose and time dependent decrease in the $\Delta\Psi_m$ for 48 h (Nigam, Bhui et al. 2009). In a similar manner Allicin in combination with 5-FU reduced mitochondrial membrane potential in human hepatocellular carcinoma (HCC) cell (Zou, Liang et al. 2016). Allicin has also shown to exhibit a loss of $\Delta\Psi_m$ in both MDA-MB-231 and MCF7 cells (Kim, Cho et al. 2016) justifying that Alliin which is converted to Allicin also modulates mitochondrial membrane potential and may be responsible for the bioactivity.

### 3.3.12 Effects of [6]-Gingerol and Alliin on Apoptotic Proteins

Insights on the mechanism underlying cell death related to apoptosis induced by [6]-Gingerol as well as Alliin was identified by changes in the level of apoptosis-related proteins. After exposure of [6]-Gingerol and Alliin on AGS cells, apoptotic protein Bax was up-regulated whereas Bcl2 was down-regulated and these alterations displaced the balance between pro- and anti-apoptotic family members on mitochondrial outer membrane towards apoptosis (Gross, McDonnell et al. 1999) which caused a loss of $\Delta\Psi_m$ and outburst of Cytochrome-c from the mitochondrial space in to the cytoplasm (Fig 3.11(A) and (B)). Cytochrome-c in the cytoplasm forms an apoptosome that in turn activates caspase-9 from its inactive state. Thereafter to accomplish the process of apoptosis, the effector Procaspases, including Procaspase 3 is activated by Caspase-9 (Zou, Yang et al. 2003). The protein level of Cytochrome-c, Caspases-9 and -3 were found to be raised by [6]-Gingerol as well as Alliin treatment in AGS cells which confirms that Caspase-9 activates Procaspase-3 to execute apoptosis. Simultaneously, treatment of AGS cells with [6]-Gingerol as well as Alliin significantly induced the release of Cytochrome c from the mitochondrial matrix which induces the caspase cascade in a dose dependent manner.

**Fig 3.11(A) Effect of [6]-Gingerol on the Expression of Apoptotic Proteins**

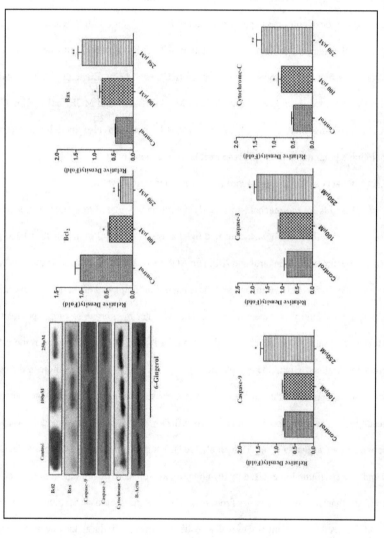

The expression levels of Bax, Bcl2, Caspase-3,9 and Cytochrome C were quantified using the computerized image analysis system Image J. Bcl2 protein levels were decreased with increase in [6]-Gingerol concentration whereas Caspase-3,9 and Cytochrome C levels were significantly increased (*$p \leq 0.05$, **$p \leq 0.01$).

## Fig 3.11(B) Effect of Alliin on the Expression of Apoptotic Proteins

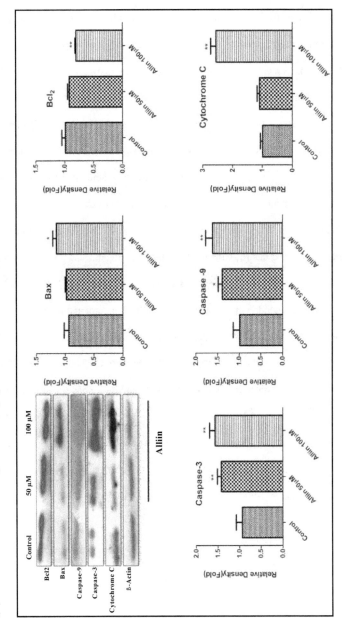

The expression levels of Bax, Bcl2, Caspase-3,9 and Cytochrome C were quantified using the computerized image analysis system Image J. Bcl2 protein levels were decreased with increase in Alliin concentration whereas Caspase-3,9 and Cytochrome C levels were significantly increased ((*p ≤ 0.05, **p ≤ 0.01).

In normal cells, Bcl2 inhibits apoptosis, which deactivates Bax by forming hetero-dimers. But, pro-apoptotic signals induce transit of Bax specifically to the mitochondria, and Bax together with Bak forms membrane-integrated homo-oligomers, which leads through the mitochondrial membrane and triggers a loss of the $\Delta\Psi_m$ subsequently leading to the release of Cytochrome-c to the cytoplasm (Chen, Guerrero et al. 2007). Inferring from previously mentioned events, the Bcl2 family proteins are pivotal players in apoptosis, especially in mitochondria-mediated apoptosis. [6]-Gingerol has been reported to induce apoptosis in A431 skin carcinoma cells by creating perturbations in Bax/Bcl2 ratio and elevation of Cytochrome-c, Caspases-9 and -3 via infliction of mitochondrial functions regulated by ROS (Nigam, Bhui et al. 2009). Recent literatures showed that [6]-Gingerol treatment activated the apoptotic pathway in osteosarcoma cells by uplifting the cleaved caspase-3, caspase-8, and caspase-9 levels (Fan, Yang et al. 2015). Likewise, mitochondria mediated apoptosis in [6]-Gingerol and Alliin treated AGS cells in the present study were because of upregulation of Bax and downregulation of Bcl2. Studies have shown that Allicin induced apoptosis of MGC-803, BGC-823 and SGC-7901 cells was mainly by elevating the expression of cleaved caspase 3 and Bax (Zhang, Zhu et al. 2015) while another report proved the apoptotic effect of Allicin on oesophageal squamous cell carcinoma (ESCC) by significant elevated level of Bax, caspase-3 and cleaved caspase-9 accompanied by Cyt c release to cytosol (Chen, Li et al. 2016). These data from the present study also suggest that executor Caspases including caspase-3 are necessary in [6]-Gingerol as well as Alliin induced occurrence of apoptosis in AGS cells. Treatment with [6]-Gingerol as well as Alliin on AGS cells facilitate activation of the extrinsic (death receptor mediated) as well as the intrinsic (mitochondrial mediated) pathway of apoptosis.

### 3.3.13 Combination Effect (Synergism) on AGS Cells

Drug combination is most efficient treatment strategies to manage dreadful diseases, like cancer and AIDS. The main aim of combining drugs is to achieve synergistic therapeutic effect wherein reduction in dose and toxicity, and minimization or delay in the induction of drug resistance can be achieved (Chou 2006). According to Chou Talaly et al, Combination Index (CI) implies the effect of multiple drug combinations (Synergism (CI<1), Additive (CI=1), Antagonism (CI>1). A mixture of moderately active metabolites present in an extract or the combination of various metabolites present in two or more drug extracts are potentially able to interfere and down regulate different proteins of the same signaling network leading to synergistic pharmacological effects (Wagner and Ulrich-Merzenich 2009) which will aid in alleviating the disease condition. In this respect, it is also convinced that *in vitro* approaches are suited for the detection of synergistic properties or pro-drugs and how important it is to follow a more holistic *in vivo* approach either via clinical trials or animal experiments (Verpoorte, Choi et al. 2005).

To check the combination effect of two drugs, cell viability assay was performed for each drug individually. In brief, $IC_{50}$ values of [6]-Gingerol and Alliin were obtained and a series of combinations at varying concentrations against cells were tested. To perform this, AGS gastric cancer cell line was exposed to various concentrations of Alliin and [6]-Gingerol at a constant ratio of 1:100. But in the case of co-treatment of aqueous ginger and garlic extract, a non-constant combination ratio of various concentrations was followed i.e. the $IC_{50}$ value of fresh ginger extract with the different values like ($IC_{30}$, $IC_{50}$, $IC_{70}$, $IC_{100}$) of fresh garlic extract and vice versa. Cell viability was assessed using MTT assay and the combination index of each combination treatment was calculated by CompuSyn software. **CompuSyn (Biosoft, UK)**, a computer software was used to analyze the dose effects for the above-mentioned combinations which first initiates with single-agent dose-response curves, followed by dose-response curves involving combinations of Alliin and [6]-Gingerol as well as fresh ginger extract with fresh garlic extract (Brahmbhatt, Gundala et al. 2013). Chou-Talalay drug combination method was followed to result in CI value. For mutually exclusive drugs exhibiting similar modes of action, the combination index is described as: **CI = (D)1/(Dx)1+(D)2/(Dx)2**, where (Dx)1 and (Dx)2 are the doses of drug 1 and drug 2 alone, respectively, causing x % inhibition, (Zhang, Zhang et al. 2017).

The drug interaction was evaluated wherein **CI value < 1 signifies synergism, =1 shows additism, or >1 confers antagonism** (Lee, Kim et al. 2014). In the case of [6]-Gingerol and Alliin interaction, combination shows moderate antagonism as shown in (Fig 3.12(A). However, it is exciting to note that the combination of aqueous ginger and garlic extract exhibits synergism as evidenced by CI<1. Points below the dotted line indicate synergy. Notably, the combined treatment of fresh ginger extract with $IC_{30}$, $IC_{50}$, $IC_{70}$, $IC_{100}$ dose of fresh garlic extract resulted in synergistic growth inhibition of AGS cells with combination index (CI) value of 0.85 as shown by combination index plot and isobologram analysis (Fig 3.12 (B)) which demonstrated that all the nine concentrations for both the drugs used lie below the black dotted line, signifying strong synergetic interaction, with CI value < 1. This probably may be the reason that Indian Culinary uses ginger-garlic paste in most of its dishes.

### 3.4 Conclusion

Ginger and garlic are two traditionally used spices, known for their medicinal values. Accordingly, in order to scientifically validate the same and identify the possible mechanism

**Fig 3.12(A) Combinatorial Effect to Check Drug Interaction ([6]-Gingerol and Alliin)**

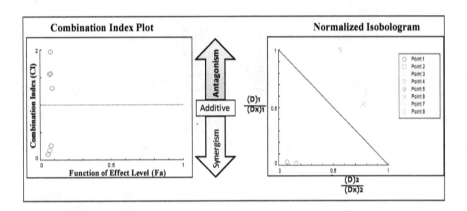

Treatment of AGS cells with a combination of [6]-Gingerol and Alliin at a fixed ratio. The antiproliferative effects were then assessed and a median effect analysis was conducted. The combination index values at the 50% fraction affected are shown (left). A normalized Isobologram profile of combined dose treatment is shown (right). Data points below, above or on the line respectively indicate synergistic, antagonistic or additive pharmacological interaction between combined treatments.

**Fig 3.12(B) Combinatorial Effect to Check Drug Interaction (Aqueous Ginger Extract and Garlic Extract)**

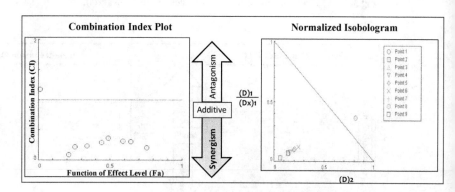

Treatment of AGS cells with a combination of ginger extract and garlic extract at a nonconstant ratio. The anti-proliferative effects were then assessed and a median effect analysis was conducted. The combination index values at the 50% fraction affected are shown (left). A normalized Isobologram profile of combined dose treatment is shown (right). Data points below, above or on the line respectively indicate synergistic, antagonistic or additive pharmacological interaction between combined treatments.

for its individual potent phytoconstituents and the whole extracts of ginger and garlic were tested on gastric adenocarcinoma cells.

- [6]-Gingerol, Alliin and the extracts of both ginger and garlic were found to possess antioxidant property which would be useful in the present-day context wherein most of the people suffer from gastric cancer related complications.
- The cytotoxicity potential of [6]-Gingerol and Alliin was found to be potent which can help to develop better cytotoxic drugs from natural origin for the treatment and management of gastric cancer.
- Further, [6]-Gingerol and Alliin elevated the percentage of early apoptotic cells in gastric adenocarcinoma cells in a dose dependent manner, which proves their anti-proliferative property. The anti-proliferative potential of [6]-Gingerol and Alliin against AGS cells was mediated by the growth arrest of cells in G2/M and S phase of cell cycle.
- Increased production of reactive oxygen species (ROS) and alteration in mitochondrial membrane potential by the treatment of [6]-Gingerol and Alliin might be responsible for triggering cytotoxicity and cell death by increasing oxidative stress in AGS cells.
- The perturbations in mitochondrial membrane potential by [6]-Gingerol and Alliin are associated with deregulation of Bax/Bcl2 ratio at protein level which leads to up-regulation of Cytochrome-c triggering the Caspase cascade in a dose dependent manner which can be effectively used for targeting the mitochondrial energy metabolism to manage gastric cancer cells.
- Concentration of [6]-Gingerol in fresh ginger extract and Alliin in fresh garlic is observed to be more than their dried extracts. Although the individual bioactive

molecules from ginger and garlic were found to be potent cytotoxic agents against AGS cells but their combination treatment exhibits a moderate antagonism.

- Interestingly a potent synergism was revealed between the co-treatment of aqueous extract of both fresh ginger and fresh garlic which prompted us to reveal the effect of individual ginger and garlic extracts and their combined synergetic effect on MNU-induced gastric cancer (*in-vivo* study).

# CHAPTER 4

## *In-Vivo Studies on the Possible Mechanism of Action of the Test Drugs*

# CHAPTER 4

## 4.1 Introduction

In the rampant increase of disease burdens, the incessant need for the development of more effective and yet less toxic drugs for the treatment of diseases such as cancer is the need of the hour. The inability to replicate the precise cellular conditions of an organism in *in vitro* studies, *in vivo* studies using whole animals/humans is preferred. Animal experimentation and human clinical trials are two distinct components of *in vivo* studies. *In vivo* testing is often employed over *in vitro* models because it is better suited for observing the overall effects of an experiment on a living organism in its natural environment as opposed to a partial or dead organism. wherein there are many reasons to believe that *in vivo* studies have the potential to offer conclusive insights and about the nature of disease. *In vivo* experiments are performed on a wide range of animal models which mimics or have near resemblance to humans and make them useful for research interpretations. One of the main advantage of performing experiments in *in vivo* model is to study the development of an organism while it is still alive and seeing how different mutations or defects affect an entire animal model. Although *in silico* and *in vitro* studies are quite popular and provides preliminary information for drug discovery, *in vivo* studies using animal models are still needed to translate and validate all the parameters in drug discovery.

Further *in vitro* studies not necessarily mimic the exact pathophysiology or natural course of any disease as they are carried out in a controlled environment with necessary supplementations. Many aspects like dietary factors and environmental conditions contribute to the pathophysiology of disease in *in vivo* conditions. As much as *in vivo* experimentations are considered, choosing appropriate animal models ensure successful understanding of the disease pathology and its mitigation. Therefore, selection of appropriate experimental animal models is the utmost necessity for fruitful bench-to-bedside translation of the therapeutic interventions. Rodents are the lowest mammals in the phylogeny wherein they possess similar genetic predispositions as humans and are easy to handle. Hence, rodent models play a major role to have a better understanding of the gene and protein functions in relation to disease conditions as well as to elucidate their molecular pathways and mechanisms (Cekanova and Rathore 2014). Cancer research involves identification of the mechanism of cancer development as well as translational research pertaining to chemoprevention and identification of specific biomarkers for early diagnosis and prognosis. In this context use of different animal models are highly exploited. There are so many animal models to induce cancer in *in vivo* experimentation such as Xenograft models, Genetically induced models and Chemical induced models.

### 4.1.1 Rodent Xenograft Cancer Model

Xenograft cancer models are constructed by transplanting cancer cells (from any origin like human or animal) in to the immunocompromised rodents either by ectopic way (under the skin) or by orthotropic way (into the organ of tumor origin) (Huynh, Abrahams et al. 2011, Ruggeri, Camp et al. 2014). Xenograft animal cancer models are the common and modest methods using cancer cell lines for generating tumors which leads to *in vivo* testing and better development of successful cancer therapy (Sharpless and DePinho 2006, Cekanova, Uddin et al. 2013). Cancer research employs a number of immunocompromised rodents like BALB/cJ, BALB/cByJ, severely compromised immune-deficient (SCID) mice and athymic nude (Forkhead box protein N1 [Foxn1nu]) mice (Morton and Houghton 2007). Athymic nude mouse is a great choice in cancer research due to the mutation of the Foxn1 gene which ultimately gives a complete failure of the immune system whereas a single nucleotide polymorphism (SNP) in the DNA-dependent protein kinase of catalytic polypeptide (Prkdc) gene in SCID rodents made them a suitable model due to its unimpaired loss of immune system. The major obstruction about xenograft rodent cancer models which limits its use in translational research is that the rats and mice used in the study do not follow the natural history of cancer due to their immunocompromised immune system, superficial vascularization of xenograft tumors, and the lack of stroma-tumor interactions (Sharpless and DePinho 2006, Frese and Tuveson 2007). Further it requires a well-established animal facility to maintain the animals and involves substantial financial cost to execute the research proposal.

### 4.1.2 Genetically Engineered Mouse Models of Cancer

Genetically engineered mouse models are the extensively used models in drug discovery and preclinical translational biology where the genome has altered through the use of genetic engineering techniques. Mostly genetically engineered models are of two types. Transgenic or Knockout mice are a type of mouse model that uses transgene with the desired sequence insertion into the pronuclei of fertilized zygotes to disrupt an existing gene's expression by replacing the gene of interest with the designed transgene through homologous recombination (Adams and Cory 1991, Dickins, McJunkin et al. 2007). Oncomice are created by inserting transgenes which helps to increase the animal's vulnerability to cancer (Thomas and Capecchi 1987). The most commonly used systems to create these models are *Cre-Lox*, tetracycline-dependent promoter regulation, and *Flp*-mediated site-specific and spontaneous recombination methods (Sauer 1987, Gossen and Bujard 1992, Schlake and Bode 1994). Cloned oncogenes carried by transgenic mice and absence of tumor suppressor genes in knockout mice are serving as potent models in cancer research (Stewart, Pattengale et al. 1984, Jacks, Fazeli et al. 1992).

However, the inability to control the level and pattern of gene expression and the expression of unwanted phenotypes due to random integration of a transgene is the major limitation of using genetically modified mouse models.

### 4.1.3 Chemically Induced Rodent Models of Cancer

Chemically induced cancer rodent models are indispensible methods which help in the study of the complex traits of cancer. Cancer burden in the human population is identified using chemically induced carcinogenesis which directly relates to the carcinogens from diet, environment and workplace. This model provides the first experimental evidence for the link between chemical exposure and cancer (Kemp 2015). Chemically induced cancer models in experimental animals can mimic the early stage of clinical cancer to the late stage which can help to better understand the molecular mechanisms involved in tumor initiation, promotion and progression, to explore the preventive measures for carcinogenesis and to evaluate the diagnostic/therapeutic effects of candidate drugs in comparison to genetically engineered cancer models and xenograft models (Liu, Yin et al. 2015). The advantages of using the chemically induced primary malignancies in mammals include the uncomplicated procedures with successive tumor generation rate and high analogy to clinical human primary cancers which can contribute to the causes and mechanism of cancer. According to the carcinogenesis potency and genotoxicity databases, nearly thirty substances such as estrogen, formaldehyde, diethylstilbestrol, DDT, vinyl chloride, neon gas, asbestos etc. first shown to cause cancer in animals are strongly associated with human cancer. Multistage chemical carcinogenesis of mouse strain is the most extensively researched animal model of cancer wherein DMBA/TPA induced mutations in the Ras oncogene and the tumor suppressor p53 shown remarkable consistency (Kemp 2015).

### 4.1.3(a) MNU-Induced Gastric Carcinogenesis

The most commonly employed carcinogens in chemically induced rodent models of gastric cancer studies are $N$-butyl-$N$-(4-hydroxybutyl)-nitrosamine, 4-(methylnitrosamino)-1-(3-pyridyl)-1-butanone, $N$-methylnitrosourea, Benzo[a]pyrene, Azoxymethane, N-nitroso-methylbenzylamine, 4,4'-nitroquinoline-1-oxide and $N$-methyl-$N$-nitro-$N$-nitrosoguanidine.

Administration of $N$-methyl-$N$-nitrosourea (MNU), a $N$-nitroso compound generated by anaerobic gut bacteria following ingestion of nitrates and nitrites is the best distinguished model of chemically induced gastric cancer. Normally MNU is administered in citrate buffer or in drinking water to induce carcinogenicity where the concentration of MNU decides its tumorigenic efficacy (Yamachika, Nakanishi et al. 1998). Most of the standard protocols recommend MNU at a concentration of 120 ppm for 5 alternating weeks or 100 mg/kg b.w. thrice a week to induce gastric cancer (Sintara K., Thong-Ngam *et al.*, 2012). A high-salt diet if provided along with MNU increases the frequency of tumor development in a significant manner (Leung, Wu et al. 2008). MNU-induced tumors occur mostly in the gastric antrum which comprise of moderately differentiated adenocarcinomas with a large stromal cell component and sometimes it is well-differentiated. The MNU-induced gastric cancer model has revealed to modulate several signaling pathways in gastric tumorigenesis which includes p53, NF-κB, mitogen-activated protein kinase (MAPK), COX-2, E-cadherin and KLF-4.

As environmental influence plays a major role in gastric cancer, MNU induced carcinogen model has been employed in the present research work so that the disease in its true nature can be observed. Based on the results of the *in vitro* studies, wherein it has been identified that synergism exists between fresh ginger and fresh garlic aqueous extract, this combination is used to carry out the animal experiment to check the in-depth efficacy evaluation and the probable mode of action in modulating MNU-induced gastric cancer.

## 4.2 Materials and Methods

### 4.2.1 Induction of Gastric Cancer

#### 4.2.1.1 Experimental Animals

5-6 weeks old male albino-Wistar rats weighing about 110-140 grams were obtained from *in vivo* Bioscience, Bengaluru and transported to the Central Animal House of Pondicherry University as per CPCSEA guidelines with IAEC approval number PU/ SLS/ AH/ IAEC/ 2016/ 04 (29.03.2016). Animals were acclimatized for one week to the experimental conditions at 24 ± 2 °C, humidity 60 ± 5% with 12 h night and day cycle in polypropylene cages. Rats were allowed standard pellet diet and drinking water *ad libitum* throughout the study.

#### 4.2.1.2 Standardization of Induction of Gastric Cancer

For induction of gastric cancer male albino Wistar rats were equally randomized in to 2 groups of eight animals each: Normal control rats (Group I) were fed with 1 mL of citrate buffer (pH - 4.5) orally and normal saline (1 mL/rat) thrice a week throughout the experiment. Cancer control rats (Group II) were administered with MNU (100 mg/kg b.w.) in citrate buffer, pH - 4.5 and normal saline thrice in a week via intragastric route initially for a period of 8 weeks and then continued till 16 weeks to check the extent of carcinogenicity. The level of cancer induction was identified by a specific biochemical marker Gastrin, oxidative stress markers Thiobarbituric acid reactive substances (TBARS) and Reduced Glutathione (GSH) confirmed by histopathological analysis.

### 4.2.1.3 Experimental Protocol and Animal Grouping for Evaluation of Protection by Drug Treatment

For induction of gastric cancer, male rats of two sets were equally randomized in to 7 groups with eight animals in each group. First set of animals were induced with MNU from $0^{th}$ week to $8^{th}$ week and drug treatment was started from $9^{th}$ week to $24^{th}$ week to evaluate the therapeutic efficacy whereas the second set of animals received MNU from $0^{th}$ week to $16^{th}$ week, with simultaneous treatment of drug from $0^{th}$ week to $24^{th}$ weeks to check the prophylactic efficacy. Normal control rats (Group I) were fed citrate buffer, pH - 4.5 (1 mL/rat) orally and normal 5% NaCl (1 mL/rat) twice a week throughout the experiment. Cancer control rats (Group II) were administrated with MNU (100 mg/kg b.w.) in citrate buffer, pH - 4.5 and 5% NaCl twice in a week via intragastric route initially for 8 weeks followed by another 8 weeks (Sintara, Thong-Ngam et al. 2012), Animals in Group III were treated with MNU and 5 Fluorouracil (40 mg/kg b.w.) once a week intraperitoneally from $9^{th}$ week to $16^{th}$ week then from $16^{th}$ week to $24^{th}$ week, Rats in Group IV as well as Group V were treated with MNU and garlic extract (100 mg/kg b.w.) and ginger extract (100 mg/kg b.w.) respectively daily by intragastric route from $9^{th}$ week to $16^{th}$ week then from $16^{th}$ week to $24^{th}$ week. Rats in Group VI were administered with MNU and garlic-ginger extract from $1^{st}$ week to $16^{th}$ week then from $16^{th}$ week to $24^{th}$ week while Rats in Group VII were given MNU and garlic-ginger extract from $9^{th}$ week to $16^{th}$ week then from $16^{th}$ week to $24^{th}$ week to identify the prophylactic and therapeutic efficacy respectively. At the end of $16^{th}$ week half of the animals from each group were fasted overnight and sacrificed to check the extent of carcinogenicity and to evaluate the effect of individual and combination of drugs on some liver toxicity markers, oxidative stress markers and on histopathology. To perform the above assays, organs (Liver and Stomach) were isolated and stored at -80 °C for biochemical analysis and a part was stored in buffered 10% formalin for the histopathological studies.

**Group I:** Control + 5% NaCl

**Group II:** Cancer control (MNU (100 mg/kg b.w.) + 5% NaCl

**Group III:** Cancer control (MNU (100 mg/kg b.w.) + 5% NaCl + 5-FU

**Group IV:** Cancer control (MNU (100 mg/kg b.w.) + 5% NaCl + Garlic Extract ($9^{th}$ week to 24 weeks)

**Group V:** Cancer control (MNU (100 mg/kg b.w.) + 5% NaCl + Ginger Extract ($9^{th}$ week to 24 weeks)

**Group VI:** Cancer control (MNU (100 mg/kg b.w.) + 5% NaCl + Ginger Garlic Extract ($1^{st}$ week to 24 weeks)

**Group VII:** Cancer control (MNU (100 mg/kg b.w.) + 5% NaCl + Ginger Garlic Extract ($9^{th}$ week to 24 weeks)

## 4.2.2 Measurement of Body Weight, Feed Intake and Water Intake of Experimental Animals

The present work identifies the influence of ginger and garlic extract individually and in combination (Prophylactic and Therapeutic dose) on MNU-induced carcinogenesis by checking the body weight, feed intake and water intake of the experimental animals throughout the study period. Weekly body weight was measured to check the health status as well as the induction of cancer whereas feed intake and water intake were measured daily for routine checkup.

### 4.2.3 Serum Biochemical Markers of Toxicity

Toxicological markers like Lactate Dehydrogenase (LDH), Alkaline Phosphatase (ALP), and Gamma Glutamyl Transferase (γGT) was measured from the serum samples of the animals collected after $16^{th}$ and $24^{th}$ week of animal experimentation. To perform the same, the animals were sacrificed under low dose of thiopental sodium anesthesia at the end of the experiment and blood was collected by sino orbital puncture. Serum was separated by centrifugation (Centrifuge 5804R, Eppendorf, Germany) at 4 °C temperature for 10 minutes at 3500 g. The serum separated was stored at -20 °C (Thermo Electron Corporation, USA) for further biochemical analysis.

#### 4.2.3.1 Estimation of Lactate Dehydrogenase

The activity of lactate dehydrogenase (LDH) was determined based on UV kinetic method. The catalytic concentration was determined from the rate of decrease of NADH measured at 340 nm.

$$\text{Pyruvate} + \text{NADH} + H^+ \xrightleftharpoons{\text{LDH}} \text{Lactate} + \text{NAD}^+$$

This enzymatic method was performed with Spinreact kit (Spain) using a semi-automated biochemical analyzer (Star 21 Plus autoanalyser, Rapid Diagnostics). The results are expressed as U/L.

#### 4.2.3.2 Estimation of Alkaline Phosphatase

Alkaline phosphatase (ALP) catalyses the transfer of the phosphate group from $p$-Nitrophenylphosphate to 2-amino-2-methyl-1-propanol (AMP), liberating $p$-Nitrophenol and the rate of $p$-Nitrophenol formation, measured is proportional to the catalytic concentration of alkaline phosphatase present in the sample which was measured at 340 nm as rate of decrease in absorbance. This enzymatic method was performed with Spinreact kit (Spain) using a semi-automated biochemical analyzer (Star 21 Plus autoanalyser, Rapid Diagnostics) and the results are expressed as U/L.

#### 4.2.3.3 Gamma Glutamyl Transferase

The activity of gamma glutamyl transferase in serum was determined based on UV – kinetic IFCC method. The color absorbs light at 405 nm and is directly proportional to the activity of GGT in serum. This enzymatic method was performed with Spinreact kit (Spain) using a semi-automated biochemical analyzer (Star 21 Plus autoanalyser, Rapid Diagnostics) and the results are expressed as U/L.

#### 4.2.3.4 Estimation of Serum Gastrin

Gastrin, a peptide hormone, which stimulates the secretion of gastric acids by the parietal cells of the stomach is a specific marker of gastric cancer. Hence, to identify the influence of its level in cancer induced rats, the level of serum gastrin was determined using a commercially available ELISA kit (Elab science, Texas) as per the manufacturer's instruction and the OD was measured at 450 nm in a microplate reader (BIO-RAD). The results are expressed as pg/mL.

#### 4.2.3.5 Estimation of C – Reactive Protein

The level of inflammatory marker C - Reactive Protein (CRP) in serum was determined using Spinreact kit method based on turbidimetric test. In this method, the CRP reacts with antihuman CRP mouse monoclonal antibody-coated latex, and agglutination occurs. CRP concentration was determined by the measurement of change in absorbance that results from the agglutination reaction.

### 4.2.4 Tissue Collection and Processing of Tissue Homogenate for Biochemical Assays

A portion of the major organs like stomach and liver from each experimental group of rats was washed with ice cold saline and was processed immediately for biochemical assays. A small representative tissue slice was stored in 10% buffered neutral formalin solution and was taken for histopathological examinations. 10% tissue homogenate of stomach and liver was prepared by adding 10% ice cold KCl solution in a homogenizer (Remi Elektrotechnik Ltd). It was centrifuged at 3500 rpm for 10 minutes and was separated into many aliquots. Each aliquot was used for specific biochemical estimations.

The enzymatic endogenous antioxidants like Glutathione Peroxidase (GPx), catalase, Glutathione-S-Tranferase (GST), Glutathione Reductase (GR) and Superoxide Dismutase (SOD); non-enzymatic endogenous antioxidants like Reduced glutathione (GSH), Vitamin C and oxidative stress markers such as thiobarbituric acid reactive substances (TBARS), ferrodoxin reducing antioxidant power (FRAP) were measured in the tissues of liver and stomach following standard procedures.

#### 4.2.4.1 Assay of Glutathione Peroxidase

**Reagents**

  i. Sodium azide (10 mM)

  ii. Glutathione (2 mM)

  iii. Hydrogen peroxide (1 mM)

  iv. TCA 10%

  v. Potassium EDTA (0.4 mM)

  vi. Tris hydrochloric acid Buffer (0.4 mM)

  vii. 2-Dinitrobenzoic acid (DTNB 0.6 mM)

**Procedure**

Glutathione peroxidase (GPx) was assayed by taking 200 µL of tris HCl buffer (0.4 M), 0.4 mM Ethylenediamine-Tetra-Acetic Acid Dipotassium ($K^+$EDTA) salt along with 100 µL of sodium azide and 200 µL of 10% homogenate (Rotruck, Pope et al. 1973). Thereafter, 200 µL of reduced glutathione solution (2 mM) was added followed by 0.1 mL of $H_2O_2$ and incubated for 10 minutes. The reaction was arrested by adding 0.5 mL of 10 % Trichloroacetic acid (TCA). The precipitate was removed by centrifugation at 4000 rpm for 10 minutes. The absorbance was read at 412 nm using a UV-spectrophotometer. The results were calculated by interpolation with the standard graph of pure glutathione (4-20 µg) and expressed as nM of GSH consumed/min/mg of protein.

### 4.2.4.2 Estimation of Catalase Activity

**Reagents**

i. Phosphate buffer (10 mM, pH 7.4)

ii. Hydrogen peroxide ($H_2O_2$)

iii. Glacial acetic acid

iv. Potassium dichromate

**Procedure**

Catalase was assayed in 200 µL of the homogenate in a final volume of 1 mL in phosphate buffer along with $H_2O_2$ (2 mM) (Sinha 1972). The reaction mixture was incubated at 37 °C for 5 minutes and then Dichromate Acetic Acid reagent (5% Potassium dichromate in water, Glacial Acetic Acid mixed in 1:3 ratio) was added to terminate the reaction and absorbance was taken at 570 nm. 2 mL Dichromate Acetic acid reagent acts as blank whereas the reaction mixture without homogenate acts as control. The catalase activity was expressed as nM/min/mg protein.

### 4.2.4.3 Assay of Glutathione $S$-Transferase

**Reagents**

i. Glutathione (1 mM)

ii. 1-chloro-2, 4-dinitrobenzene (CDNB) (1 mM in ethanol)

iii. Phosphate buffer (0.1 M, pH 6.5)

**Procedure**

Glutathione $S$-transferase activity was assayed with 0.1 mL of GSH, 0.1 mL of CDNB and phosphate buffer in a total volume of 2.9 mL (Habig, Pabst et al. 1974). The reaction was initiated by the addition of 0.1 mL of the 10% homogenate. The readings were recorded every 15 seconds at 340 nm against distilled water blank for a minimum of three minutes in a spectrophotometer. The assay mixture without the homogenate served as the control to monitor nonspecific binding of the substrates. The result of glutathione $S$-transferase activity was expressed in nM/min/mg Protein.

### 4.2.4.4 Assay of Glutathione Reductase

**Reagents**

i. Potassium phosphate buffer (0.2 M), pH-7.0 containing 2 mM EDTA

ii. 2 mM NADPH in 10 mM Tris-HCl buffer, pH-7.0

iii. 20 mM oxidized glutathione (GSSG)

**Procedure**

Glutathione Reductase was assayed in 0.5 mL of phosphate buffer, 50 µL GSSG and deionized water to make a total volume of 1 mL (Staal, Visser et al. 1969). The reaction was initiated by the addition of 200 µL of 10% tissue homogenate. The change in absorbance at 340 nm was followed at 30 °C for every minute for 5 minute. Values are expressed as nM/min/mg Protein.

### 4.2.4.5 Assay of Superoxide Dismutase

**Reagents**

    i. Sodium pyrophosphate buffer (0.025 M, pH 7.4)

    ii. Phenazonium Metho Sulphate (PMS) (186 µM)

    iii. Nitro Blue Tetrazolium chloride (NBT) (300 µM)

    iv. NADH (780 µM)

    v. Glacial acetic acid

    vi. n-Butanol

**Procedure**

Superoxide dismutase was assayed by taking 50 µL of 10% tissue homogenate followed by addition of 0.3 mL of sodium pyrophosphate buffer, 0.025 mL of PMS and 0.075 mL of NBT (Kakkar, Das et al. 1984). The reaction was started by addition of 0.075 mL of NADH. After incubation at 30 °C for 90 seconds, the reaction was stopped by addition of 0.25 mL glacial acetic acid. Then the reaction mixture was stirred vigorously and shaken with 2.0 mL of n-butanol. The mixture could stand for 10 minutes followed by centrifugation. The color intensity of the chromogen was read at 560 nm. Results were expressed as Unit/ min/mg protein.

### 4.2.4.6 Estimation of Thiobarbituric Acid Reactive Substances

**Reagents**

    i. Thiobarbituric acid (TBA) 0.8% in 0.5 N hydrochloric acid

    ii. Butylated hydroxyl toluene (BHT) 0.05% in methanol.

iii. Saline

**Procedure**

The method was initiated by heating the tissue homogenate with 0.8 mL saline, 0.5 mL of butylated hydroxy toluene and 3.5 mL thiobarbituric acid reagent for 90 seconds in a boiling water bath (Ohkawa, Ohishi et al. 1979). After cooling, the solution was centrifuged at 2,000 rpm for 10 minutes to remove the precipitate. The absorbance of the supernatant was determined at 532 nm using a spectrophotometer against a blank that contained all the reagents except the tissue homogenate. The results were calculated by interpolation with the standard malondialdehyde and the levels of TBARS are expressed as µmoles/mg tissue.

### 4.2.4.7 Ferrodoxin Reducing Antioxidant Power Assay

**Reagents**

i. Acetate buffer (300 mM, pH 3.6)

ii. TPTZ ((2, 4, 6-tripyridyl- s- triazine) in 40 mM HCl)

iii. $FeCl_3 \cdot 6H_2O$

iv. FRAP reagent (i: ii: iii in the ratio of 10:1:1)

**Procedure**

The assay was initiated by 100 µL tissue homogenate with 3 mL of working FRAP reagent and the absorbance was measured at 593 nm after thorough vortexing of the reaction mixture (Benzie and Strain 1996). Calculation was done through regression analysis by preparing standard curve of ascorbic acid. The reducing power was expressed as µg/mL of $FeSO_4$.

### 4.2.4.8 Estimation of Reduced Glutathione

**Reagents**

   i. TCA 5%

   ii. Phosphate buffer (0.2 M, pH 8)

   iii. 5,5-dithio-bis-(2-nitrobenzoic acid) (DTNB-0.6 mM) in phosphate buffer.

**Procedure**

Glutathione content was estimated in 0.25 mL of 10 % tissue homogenate by the addition of equal volume of ice cold 5 % TCA and allowed for centrifugation at 4000 rpm for 10 minutes. Thereafter 0.25 mL of phosphate buffer and 0.5 mL of DTNB was added to 1 mL of supernatant and mixed well. The absorbance was read at 412 nm using a spectrophotometer. The results were calculated by interpolation with the pure glutathione and expressed as µmoles of GSH present /mg tissue (Ellman 1959).

### 4.2.4.9 Assay of Vitamin C

**Reagents**

   i. 10 % (W/V) TCA

   ii. 65 % (V/V) $H_2SO_4$

   iii. DNPH-thiourea-copper sulphate reagent (DTC): This contains 0.4 g thiourea, 0.05 g copper sulphate and 3 g DNPH in 100 mL of 9N $H_2SO_4$

   iv. Stock standard: 100 mg L-ascorbic acid in 5 % TCA

**Procedure**

Vitamin C was assayed with 0.5 mL of the tissue homogenate incubated with 1.5 mL of ice-cold TCA followed by centrifugation at 4000 rpm for 10 minutes. 0.1 mL DTC reagent was added to 0.5 mL of supernatant, mixed well and incubated for 37 °C for 3 h (Omaye, Turnbull et al. 1979). 0.75 mL of ice-cold 65% $H_2SO_4$ was added to this mixture followed by an additional incubation for 30 minutes. Standard ascorbic acid was also processed in the same manner. The absorbance was read at 520 nm by keeping a blank of 0.5 mL TCA and the amount of ascorbic acid is expressed as μM/mg tissue.

### 4.2.4.10 Estimation of Total Protein

**Reagents**

i. Sodium carbonate (2 %) in 0.1 N sodium hydroxide (Reagent A)

ii. Copper sulphate (0.5 %) in 1% potassium sodium tartrate (Reagent B).

iii. Alkaline copper sulphate: Mixture of 50 mL of A and 1 mL of B prior to use (Reagent C)

iv. Folin – Ciocalteau reagent (Reagent D): commercially available (1:2 dilution)

v. Stock Protein solution: 10 mg of bovine serum albumin (fraction V) dissolve in distilled water and made up to 10 mL in a volumetric flask.

vi. Working standard: Dilute 1 mL of the stock solution to 5 mL with distilled water in a volumetric flask. (Conc: 0.2 mg/mL).

**Procedure**

50 μL of tissue homogenate was made to 1 mL with distilled water in a test tube. 1 mL of reagent C was added to each tube including the blank (1 mL of water) mixed well and kept for incubation for 10 minutes (Lowry et al., 1951). After incubation 0.1 mL of reagent D was added and incubated at room temp in the dark for 30 minutes. Thereafter the absorbance of blue color developed was measured at 660 nm. The protein content of both the stomach and liver tissues were determined from the standard graph of BSA.

### 4.2.5 Gene Expression Studies

#### 4.2.5.1 RNA Isolation and cDNA Synthesis

A homogeneous lysate of the frozen tissues was prepared by lysing with 1 mL of TRI reagent through firm grinding. Lysate was kept for 15 minutes in room temperature to which 200 µL of chloroform was added and vortexed well. Thereafter, centrifugation under 12000 g for 15 minutes at 4 °C was carried out to separate the aqueous and organic layers. The aqueous layer which contains RNA was pelleted by centrifugation under 12000 g for 10 minutes at 8 °C with addition of 500 µL of 2-proponal. Pellet obtained was washed with 1 mL of 70% ethanol followed by vortexing for three times and centrifugation was performed under 7500 g for 5 minutes at 4 °C.

Finally, isolated total RNA was suspended in RNAase free water (Chomczynski and Mackey 1995) and quantified using a Nano drop. Briefly, 1 µL of total RNA isolated was placed on Nano drop which analyses the samples at 260 nm/280 nm and 260 nm/230 nm. Concentration of RNA was adjusted to contain 2 µg/mL uniformly in all the samples and cDNA was synthesized using a kit (High cDNA, Applied biosystem) as per the manufacture's instruction by employing random primers, reverse transcriptase and dNTPs suspended in buffer.

#### 4.2.5.2 Real Time PCR

Quantitative real time PCR (qPCR) amplifications were performed in triplicate using an ABI prism™ 7700 sequence detection system (Applied biosystems). Reaction mixture contains 1 µL of template (cDNA), 300 nM each of forward and reverse primers and 1x SYBR green PCR master mix (Applied Biosystems). The pre-denaturation condition for RT-PCR was kept at 95°C for 30s, denaturation at 95 °C for 5s and Annealing for 55 °C for 10s and the amplification was done for 40 cycles. The changes in fluorescence of SYBR green dye in every cycle were monitored, and threshold cycle (ct) above background for each reaction was calculated. Expression of genes was expressed in terms of fold change in comparison to the ct of housekeeping gene B-actin (Bonetta 2005).

#### 4.2.5.2a Estimation of Oxidative Stress Markers

The expression of Thioredoxin and Glutaredoxin which are the major markers of antioxidant system was studied in stomach tissue of the MNU-induced gastric carcinoma rats and after treatment with individual drugs and the combination of drugs. The mRNA levels of the encoded genes were checked using quantitative RT-PCR (i.e. $24^{th}$ week). The primer sequence is as follows.

| | |
|---|---|
| **TRX F:** | 5'-GGT GGA CTT CTC TGC TAC G3' |
| **TRX R:** | 5'-AAA ACT GGA AGG TCG GCA T3' |
| **GRX F:** | 5'-TGT TCA TCA AGC CCA CCT G3' |
| **GRX R:** | 5'-AGT CAT CAG CTC CCC AGT C3' |

#### 4.2.5.2b Estimation of Inflammatory Markers

Inflammation is a major pathology in cancerous lesions. Hence, to determine the role of ginger extract, garlic extract and their combination on inflammation, the gene expression of the pro-inflammatory markers such as NF-kB, TNF-α, IL-6, IL-2, COX-2 and PGE2 in MNU-induced gastric cancer was performed in the stomach tissue of the experimental animals (i.e. $24^{th}$ week). The primer sequence is as follows.

| | |
|---|---|
| **IL-2 F:** | 5'ATG ATG CTT TGA CAG ATG3' |
| **IL-2 R:** | 5'AGC GTG TGT TGG ATT TGA3' |
| **IL-6 F:** | 5'GCC TTC TTG GGA CTG ATG3' |
| **IL-6 R:** | 5'GGT CTG TTG TGG GTG GTA3' |

| | |
|---|---|
| IL-10 F: | 5'ATAACTGCACCCACTTCCCA3' |
| IL-10 R: | 5'TTTCTGGGCCATGGTTCTCT3' |
| TNFα F: | 5'GAC CCC TTT ACT CTG ACC CC3' |
| TNFα R: | 5'ACC TGA CCA CTC TCC CTT TG3' |
| PGE2 F: | 5'GAC CAG GCA TTG TGT GAC3' |
| PGE2 R: | 5'AGA AGT AGG CGT GGT TGA3' |
| COX-2F: | 5'CAGGTCATCGGTGGAGAG3' |
| COX-2R: | 5'CTCGTCATCCCACTCAGG3' |
| NfkB F: | 5'CAC CAA AGA CCC ACC TCA3' |
| NfkB R: | 5'GGA CCG CAT TCA AGT CAT3' |
| B-actin F: | 5'ATG GAG AAG ATT TGG CAC C3' |
| B-actin R: | 5'GGT CAT CTT TTC ACG GTTG 3' |

### 4.2.6 Protein Expression Studies by Western Blot

**Reagents**

i. RIPA buffer

ii. Laemmli 2X buffer/loading buffer (125 mM Tris-HCl, pH - 6.8, 4% SDS, 20% Glycerol, 10% β-mercaptoethanol and 0.004% bromophenol blue)

iii. Running buffer (0.25 M Tris, 0.5%- SDS, 1.92 M Glycine)

iv. Transfer buffer

v. Blocking buffer (5% non-fat dry milk powder and 0.1% Tween 20 in 1X TBS)

vi. 1X Tris buffered Saline (TBS), pH 7.4 (0.2 M Tris in 0.89% NaCl)

vii. Ponceau stain (0.1% ponceau in 1% acetic acid)

viii. Antibody dilution buffer (5% BSA, 0.1% Tween-20 in 1X TBS

**Procedure**

Stomach tissues of control and experimental groups of rats (i.e. 24$^{th}$ week) were homogenized in 135 mM NaCl, 20 mM Tris, 2 mM EDTA and 1 mM PMSF (pH 7.4). The homogenates were centrifuged at 12000 g at 4 °C for 15 minutes and the concentration of the total protein was determined from the supernatant by Lowry method. Then equal amount of protein (50 µg) was resolved on a 12% SDS-Polyacrylamide gel for electrophoresis and then transferred to PVDF membrane by a semidry transfer unit (Hoefer). Membranes were blocked with Tris buffered saline (TBS) containing 5% non-fat dry milk for 2 h to avoid non-specific binding sites and incubated with 1:1000 dilution of primary antibodies (B-Actin, Caspase-9, Caspase-3, Bax, Bcl2 and Cytochrome-c from Santa cruz) overnight, and then washed with TBS containing 0.1% Tween-20 and incubated with HRP-conjugated secondary antibody at 1:2500 dilution for 90 minutes at room temperature (Towbin, Staehelin et al. 1979). After proper washing with TBS containing 0.1% Tween-20 for three times, the transferred proteins were visualized on X-ray photographic film and quantified by Image J software.

### 4.2.7 Histopathological Analysis

**Reagents**

i. 10 % buffered neutral formalin

ii. Hematoxylin and Eosin stain (Lillie Mayer alum preparation): Aluminium ammonium sulphate (200 g), haematoxylin (20 g), ethanol (40 mL), sodium iodate (4 g), acetic acid (80 mL), glycerol (1200 ml) were mixed well with distilled water (2800 mL).

iii. Acetified eosin/phloxine 1% eosin (400 mL), 1% aqueous phloxine (40 mL), 95% alcohol (3100 mL and glacial acetic acid (16 mL)

iv. Absolute alcohol.

v. Acid alcohol 0.3%: Ethanol (2800 mL), distilled water (1200 mL), hydrochloric acid (12 mL)

vi. Scott's tap water substitute: Sodium hydrogen carbonate (10 gm), magnesium sulphate (100 gm) and distilled water (5 L)

**Procedure**

To study the histopathological changes, the stomach tissues were collected from all the animals dissected, washed thoroughly with ice cold saline and preserved in 10 % buffered neutral formalin. Tissues were embedded in paraffin wax, sectioned to 5-7 mm thickness and fixed on glass slides. Removal of paraffin wax was done by heating the sections on water bath followed by air drying for dehydration. Staining was performed with the haematoxylin stain followed by a brief rinse in running tap water, differentiated with 0.3% acid alcohol and finally rinsed with tap water. Thereafter, sections were rinsed in Scott's tap water substitute and again washed in tap water. Counter staining with eosin was done for 2 minutes followed by rinse as well as dehydration. Finely stained sections were then mounted on coverslip with DPX agent [IHC world protocols – H and E staining]. They were examined under a light microscope. All deviations from normal histology were recorded and compared with the corresponding controls.

### 4.2.8 Statistical Analysis

The results of all data for *in-vivo* studies (Toxicological markers, Enzymatic and nonenzymatic antioxidants of liver and stomach) were statistically evaluated and analyzed through two-way Analysis of Variance (ANOVA) followed by Bonferroni multiple comparison test while the gene expression studies and immunoblot quantification were analyzed through one-way Analysis of Variance followed by Tukey's multiple comparison test respectively. They were evaluated by Graph pad prism software (version 5.0) and the results were expressed as

Mean ± SEM for eight rats in each group and a value of (p ≤ 0.05), (p ≤ 0.01) and (p ≤ 0.001) was considered significant.

## 4.3 Results and Discussion

Although, various animal models exist for gastric cancer like induction with $N$-nitrosodiethylamine, $N$-methyl-$N$-nitro-$N$-nitrosoguanidine, Benzo[a]pyrene, $N$-Methyl-$N$-nitrosurea and genetic models C57/Bl6, C3H/HeN and Sprague dawley rats to screen anti-cancer drugs, still they are encountered with some limitations. $N$-methyl-$N$-nitrosourea, a alkylating agent and a $N$-nitroso compound which induces mutation specifically through AT:GC transition is considered as the best characterized model for chemical induced gastric cancer (Poh, O'donoghue et al. 2016). Induction of gastric carcinomas by $N$-methyl-$N$-nitrosourea (MNU) in male rats is one of the most frequently used animal models for the investigation of stomach carcinogenesis and tumor treatment due to the several advantages it possesses, such as reliability of tumor induction, organ site specificity and predominantly carcinomatous histopathologic characterization, and the ability to examine tumor initiation and promotion processes. A high-salt diet if provided along with MNU increases the frequency of tumor development in a significant manner (Yamamoto, Furihata et al. 2002, Leung, Wu et al. 2008). So, a model was proposed by injecting a dose of 100 mg/kg b.w. of MNU followed by 5% NaCl in drinking water to accomplish this study. From the etiological point of view, increased consumption of salty, smoked and fried foods which are not nutritious along with the sedentary life style is the ingenious factor of gastric cancer in recent years. Hence, studying the anti-carcinogenic efficacy of the test drug in the proposed animal model creating gastric cancer in humans is more appropriate.

Results of the present study were compared with an allopathic as well as antimetabolite drug 5-Flurouracil, a fluorinated derivative of pyrimidine uracil whose mechanism of cytotoxicity is based on the inhibition of thymidylate synthase, a nucleotide synthetic enzyme in DNA replication and mis-incorporation of fluoronucleotides into RNA and DNA (Longley, Harkin et al. 2003). 5-FU-based chemotherapy proved to exhibit great impact in curing colorectal cancer (Labianca, Marsoni et al. 1995). The efficiency of two common used spices *Zingiber officinale* and *Allium sativum* individually and in combination against gastric cancer is discussed under various headings such as anti-inflammatory activity, anti-oxidant potency; role on apoptosis related proteins, biomarkers of gastro-intestinal condition and on toxicological parameters thereby scientifically authenticating the traditional claim.

### 4.3.1 Standardization of Gastric Cancer Induction by MNU

To check the extent of carcinogenicity, preliminary study was carried out to identify the induction of gastric cancer by MNU in the experimental rats by observing the changes in the biochemical and histopathology parameters as well as a specific marker of gastric cancer-Gastrin for two time periods namely $8^{th}$ week and $16^{th}$ week. As cancer is a condition of three stages like initiation, promotion and progression hence, dose duration finding study was undertaken for studying the carcinogenicity of MNU in male albino Wistar rats regarding dose and time of exposure. The experimental protocol for the whole animal experimentation is presented in Fig 4.1.

#### 4.3.1.1 Tissue Biochemical Markers

#### 4.3.1.1a Tissue TBARS Level

Generation of reactive oxygen species (ROS) which are highly reactive and unstable oxygen containing molecules occurs in excess during chemical carcinogenesis metabolism.

## Fig 4.1 Experimental Protocol for Animal Study

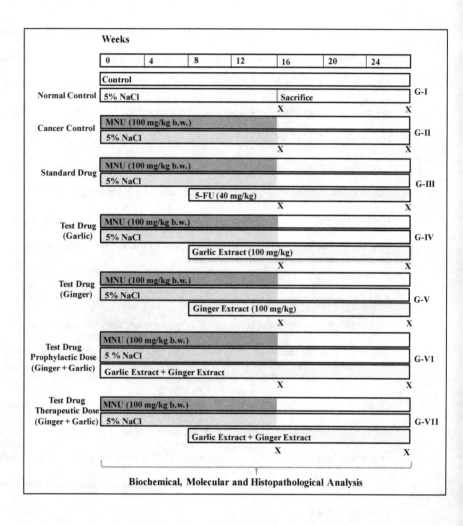

ROS can react and damage cellular macromolecules like proteins, DNA etc. ROS are the key players in carcinogenesis due to their mutagenic oxidation of DNA. MNU, a chemical carcinogen gets metabolized to different nitrate ions, diazomethanes and generates free radicals that may contribute to the initiation of lipid peroxidation (LPO). Malondialdehyde an important byproduct measured as TBARS is accepted as an indicator of LPO and is reported to be higher in cancer tissues than in non-diseased organ (Nielsen, Mikkelsen et al. 1997, Marnett 1999) Therefore, in the present study, lipid peroxidation is used as a marker to detect the extent of carcinogenicity in both 8 weeks and 16 weeks duration of MNU administration. Although cancer control rats showed a significant increase in TBARS level in comparison to normal rats in both 8 weeks ($p \leq 0.05$) and 16 weeks ($p \leq 0.01$) of MNU induction, the TBARS level in 16 weeks of MNU induction is 2.5-fold higher in comparison to the level in 8 weeks (Fig 4.2(A)). The increased level of lipid peroxidation in gastric tissues of MNU-induced rats confirms involvement of oxidative stress in MNU-induced gastric cancer when compared with group 1 normal controls. Hence, based on the results, 100 mg/kg b.w. of MNU for 8 weeks as well as 16 weeks was used in male rats to induce gastric cancer

#### 4.3.1.1b  Tissue Reduced Glutathione Level

The most important endogenous defense system against oxidative stress is the glutathione system whose major function includes cell differentiation, proliferation, and apoptosis and detoxification of xenobiotics and some endogenous compounds. Disturbances in GSH homeostasis leads to an increased susceptibility to oxidative stress implicated in the progression of cancer (Traverso, Ricciarelli et al. 2013). Many diseases such as cancer, heart attack, stroke and diabetes have been reported to have a decreased glutathione level (Wu, Fang et al. 2004). Hence, the activity of GSH content is critical for the survival of cells. In the present study, the stomach GSH levels of male rats depleted significantly ($p \leq 0.01$) on MNU induction when compared to the normal rats in both 8 weeks ($p \leq 0.05$) and 16 weeks ($p \leq 0.01$) exposure (Fig 4.2(B)). Low levels of GSH observed in the MNU-induced rats may be due to the tissue response to oxidative stress during carcinogenesis and further confirms the induction of lesions of gastric cancer.

### 4.3.1.2 Effect of MNU on Gastrin-Marker of Gastric Cancer

Gastrin is a peptide hormone secreted in the gastric mucosa. It is involved in the pathogenesis of gastric cancer and hypergastrinoma which leads to gastric carcinogenesis (Waldum, Sagatun et al. 2017). Patients with differentiated cancer and duodenal ulcer showed a significant negative correlation between gastric acid secretion and age, but it had a significant positive correlation between serum gastrin levels and age (Ferrand and Wang 2006). In this study, we found a significant increase in gastrin level ($p \leq 0.01$) in serum of cancer control rats which confirms a relationship between the positive effects of gastrin on cell growth and tumour progression in cancer (Tsukamoto, Mizoshita et al. 2015). In the present study, serum gastrin levels of normal control group after 8 weeks and 16 weeks was found to be $155 \pm 10.58$ pg/mL and $168 \pm 12$ pg/mL respectively whereas the mean serum gastrin level of MNU induced cancer rats were found to be $419.24 \pm 28.47$ and $653.24 \pm 32.47$ in the $8^{th}$ and $16^{th}$ week of cancer induction respectively (Fig 4.2(C)). The gastrin level of cancer control animals in the $16^{th}$ week was found to increase 1.5-fold in comparison to the $8^{th}$ week animals confirming the progression of cancerous lesions. Although it is obvious that the gastrin level, a specific marker of gastric carcinogenesis is significantly increased ($p \leq 0.01$) in both $8^{th}$ and $16^{th}$ week of MNU along with 5 % NaCl induction in comparison to the normal animals, it is interesting to note that there is considerable difference in the gastrin level i.e. 2.7-fold and 3.8-fold increase as compared to

## Fig 4.2 Effect of MNU on Gastric Cancer Induced Experimental Animals

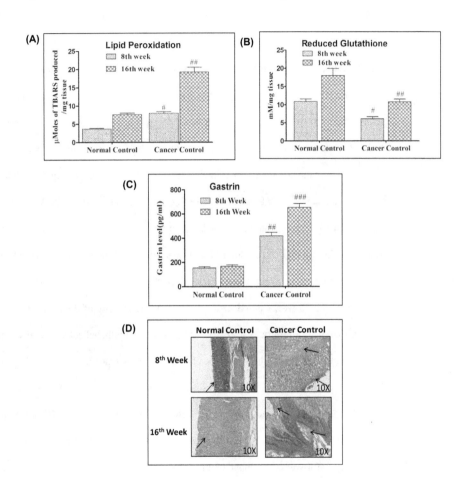

Lipid peroxidation (A), Reduced glutathione (B), Gastrin (C) and histopathology view of gastric mucosa (D) of experimental animals for 8 weeks and 16 weeks. Results are expressed in Mean ± SEM, n = 8 animals/group. Statistical analysis was performed using two tailed unpaired t tests. #, ##, ### indicates p value ≤ 0.05 and 0.01, 0.001 respectively vs control rat.

normal rats in the 8$^{th}$ and 16$^{th}$ week of carcinogenesis respectively. Accordingly, it can be confirmed that the different stages of carcinogenesis namely initiation, promotion and progression is identified.

### 4.3.1.3 Effect of MNU on Histopathological Changes of Gastric Mucosa

The MNU-induced carcinogenicity was further confirmed by histopathological analysis. Histopathological alterations in stomach tissue both for 8 weeks and 16 weeks were observed in MNU-induced male rats. Herein in the present study, control animals possessed normal keratinization in the non-glandular epithelium likewise the glandular stomach exhibited normal mucosa and glands in both 8 and 16 weeks of cancer induction whereas the MNU induced rats disclosed that the non-glandular stomach epithelium was hypertrophic with vacuolations and orthokeratotic hyperkeratosis after 16 weeks of MNU-induction but vaculations and hyperkeartosis was not that much observed at 8 weeks of MNU-induction (Fig 4.2(D)). However, in the 16 weeks intoxicated rat stomach, the severity of the damage was high and severe inflammatory infiltrates with swollen and necrotic epithelial cells were observed.

From the results of the study it can be concluded that gastric cancer was induced in rats within 16 weeks. As evidenced by the biochemical markers (Gastrin, LPO and GSH), it was found that gastric cancer was induced at a dose of 100 mg/kg b.w. of MNU and 5 % NaCl in drinking water in 16 weeks although the gastric lesions with complications has already initiated in the period of 8 weeks. Histopathological findings in the stomach tissue of cancer animals revealed a severity of cancerous lesions observed in 16 weeks in comparison to 8 weeks. The severities of the alterations were high in 16 weeks compared to that of 8 weeks exposed rats.

Based on the above justification MNU with 5 % NaCl in drinking water was employed in male rats for 8 weeks as well as 16 weeks to compare the status of different biochemical parameters, toxicological markers at a dose of 100 mg/kg b.w. and to determine the efficacy of ginger, garlic and the combination effect of both spices in ameliorating the carcinogenic effects of MNU.

### 4.3.2 Evaluation of Anticancer Potential of Test Drugs

#### 4.3.2.1 Measurement of Body Weight, Water and Feed Intake

Based on the standardization of induction of MNU-induced gastric cancer in the experimental animals, the efficacy of ginger, garlic and the combination effect (prophylactic and therapeutic dose) in ameliorating the carcinogenicity of MNU was studied in detail. The present work affirms the effect of MNU on body weight, feed intake and water intake of experimental animals in the various groups (Fig 4.3). $N$-nitroso-$N$-methylurea has been studied in mutagenicity and genetic studies to induce different types of cancer (Pubchem, chemistry database, NCBI). As every disease has its own early signs and symptoms, gastric cancer also shows symptoms like heartburn, upper abdominal pain, nausea, difficulty in swallowing, loss of appetite and finally weight loss. In our study, there was a significant decrease in bodyweight ($p \leq 0.01$) as well as feed intake in cancer induced rats compared to normal control rats. Oral gavage of the test drugs substantially increased the body weight (Fig 4.3(A)) and feed intake (Fig 4.3(B)) in comparison to the cancer control rats. Likewise, a significant decrease in water intake (Fig 4.3(C)) has been observed ($p \leq 0.001$) in cancer control rats compared to garlic extract, ginger extract treated rats, combination effect of garlic and ginger and 5-FU treated rats as well. The marked weight loss observed in cancer-bearing rats could be related to cancer cachexia or anorexia (Tisdale 2001) which leads to progressive skeletal muscle wasting. The inflammatory change related to ulceration in the stomach of cancer-induced rats may lead to loss of appetite which might result in decrease in body weight (Nicolini, Ferrari et al. 2013). The mean increase in body weight in the present study upon simultaneous administration of combination effect of garlic and ginger extract might be due to the preventive potency of bioactive phytocompounds of garlic (Omar and Al-Wabel 2010, Yun, Ban et al. 2014) and excellent cancer preventive potential of ginger owing to its antioxidant and anti-inflammatory activity (Shukla and Singh 2007).

### 4.3.2.2 Protective Effect of Test Drugs on Biochemical Markers in Serum

The protective effect of garlic extract, ginger extract and the combination effect of garlic and ginger was quantitatively assessed through various biochemical markers like ALP, γ-GT, LDH, CRP and gastrin level which are sensitive indicators of damage of cellular tissue. Enzymes such as alkaline phosphatase (ALP), Glutamyl transferase (γ-GT) and lactate dehydrogenase (LDH) are considered as diagnostic markers for normal liver functioning (Chatterjee, Patel et al. 2002). Immunological, metabolic or any other insult to the tissues and organs causes elevation of these enzymes in blood. Cancer also disturbs the level of these enzymes (Guo, Sun et al. 2003). The present data represented in (Fig 4.4(A)) exhibits a significant increase of ALP ($p \leq 0.01$) activity in serum of cancer induced rats in both $16^{th}$ week and $24^{th}$ week of drug treatment compared to the normal control group. Our results are in line with earlier reports of increased ALP isoenzymes in carcinoma of rat stomach induced by nitroso carcinogenic agent (Miki, Oda et al. 1980). LDH is a redox enzyme often overexpressed in gastric cancer permitting its survival in stressful tumor environment (Kolev, Uetake et al. 2008). Increased activity of LDH as observed in in MNU-induced rats is possibly because of damage of both the gastrointestinal tissue and liver tissue (Fig 4.4(B)). Garlic extract, ginger extract and the combination of garlic and ginger extract and 5-FU treated rats exhibited reduced LDH activity both in both the $16^{th}$ week and $24^{th}$ week of drug treatment possibly due to its protective effect. It is impressive to

**Fig 4.3 Effect of Test Drugs on Different Physiological Parameters**

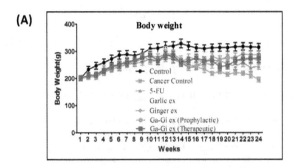

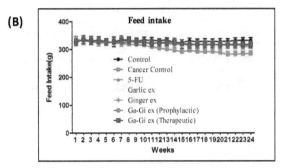

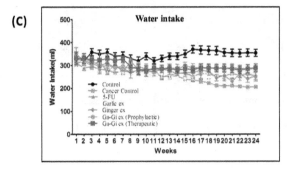

Body weight (A), feed intake (B) and water intake (C) changes in experimental animals till complete experiment. Results are expressed in Mean ± SEM, n = 8 animals/group. Statistical analysis was performed using one way ANOVA followed by Tukey's multiple comparison test. ## indicates p value ≤ 0.01 vs normal rat, *, ** indicates p value ≤ 0.05 and 0.01, respectively vs cancer control rat.

note that the combination of ginger and garlic modulated the LDH leakage both prophylactically and therapeutically. However, a decrease in γ-GT activity was observed in serum ($p \leq 0.05$) of cancer control rat when compared to normal rats (Fig 4.4(C)) which clearly shows that γ-GT is not a specific marker of stomach lesions but characteristic of liver damage and hence not associated to stomach cancer. The administration of combination of ginger and garlic extract both prophylactically and therapeutically exhibit significant elevated level ($p \leq 0.01$) only in $24^{th}$ week.

Gastrin, a peptide hormone stimulates the secretion of gastric acid by parietal cells of stomach and further stimulates the smooth muscle contraction and water secretion in stomach. A significant level of gastrin may be an indicator of severe cancerous condition. Although CA 72-4, CEA, CA 19-9, Alpha-fetoprotein are indicators for advanced gastric cancer, and postoperatively their serum levels may decrease considerably, there is a close correlation between Gastrin and gastric adenocarcinoma in clinical practice which might be of great value for the diagnosis in early stage of gastric cancer (Mattar, Andrade et al. 2002). In the present study, the serum gastrin level for cancer control group is high ($633.24 \pm 30.47$) after 16 weeks and ($876.24 \pm 42.47$) after 24 weeks in comparison to their respective normal rats. whereas the ginger extract, garlic extract and the combination of ginger and garlic extract administered rats (prophylactic and therapeutic) group showed a significant ($p \leq 0.01$) 3-fold decrease in mean serum gastrin level after 16 weeks and a 4-fold decrease after 24 weeks compared to the MNU-induced rats which is surprisingly better than the mean serum gastrin level in 5-FU group in both 16 weeks and 24 weeks of animal experimentation. Fig 4.5(A) depicts the mean serum gastrin level of all the experimental groups in both 16- and 24 weeks of drug treatment.

**Fig 4.4 Effect of Test Drugs on Serum Biochemical Markers of Toxicity**

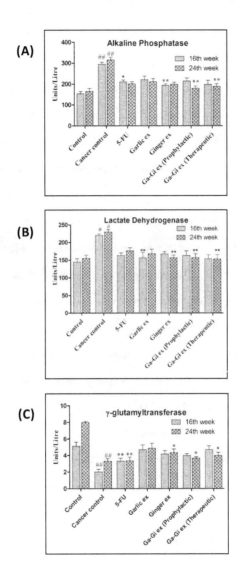

Alkaline Phosphatase (A), Lactate Dehydrogenase (B), and γ-Glutamyltransferase (C) of experimental animals for 16 weeks and 24 weeks. Results are expressed in Mean ± SEM, n = 8 animals/group. Statistical analysis was performed by using two-way Analysis of Variance (ANOVA) using graph pad prism software followed by Bonferroni multiple comparison test. # indicates p value ≤ 0.05, ## indicates p value ≤ 0.01 vs normal rat, *, ** and *** indicates p value ≤ 0.05, 0.01 and 0.001 respectively vs cancer control rat.

C-reactive protein (CRP), an acute phase protein, synthesized by hepatocytes which perform anti-infection function in the immune system and chronic inflammation involved with malignancies is considered as a marker for inflammatory conditions related to cancer (Kim, Oh et al. 2009). Invasive cancer shows higher serum CRP levels than in cases of non-invasive cancer (Polterauer, Grimm et al. 2007, Nozoe, Mori et al. 2008). In the present study, the MNU alone challenged rats showed a significant two-fold increase in CRP than the normal rats in both 16 weeks and 24 weeks (Fig 4.5(B)), whereas ginger extract, garlic extract and mostly the combination of ginger and garlic extract administered rats (prophylactic and therapeutic dose) displayed a decreased level indicating their suppression of proinflammatory cytokines and their hepatoprotectivity. The proinflammatory response in the liver results in the increased secretion of IL $-1\beta$ and TNF-$\alpha$ which in turn releases IL-6 which then stimulates the liver to secrete CRP. Therefore, it is described as a bystander marker of inflammation, having an indirect role in the inflammatory process (Rani, Madhavi et al. 2006). Based on the results of some enzymatic markers in the present study, it is evident that combination of ginger and garlic extract both prophylactically and therapeutically alleviate the damage caused by gastric cancer induced by MNU in a conspicuous manner.

### 4.3.3 Anti-Oxidant Efficacy of Test Drugs

#### 4.3.3.1 Biochemical Markers of Oxidative Stress (TBARS, FRAP)

Oxidative stress caused due to an imbalance between ROS generation and antioxidants depletion or down regulation of ROS scavengers is associated with various human diseases including many cancers. Central cellular processes such as proliferation, apoptosis, senescence are influenced by ROS and leads to the development of cancer (Waris and Ahsan 2006). Oxidative stress associated with increased levels of LPO and other thiobarbituric acid reactive

**Fig 4.5 Effect of Test Drugs on Some Specific Markers of Gastric Cancer**

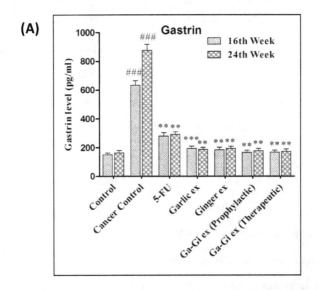

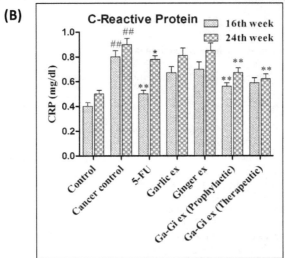

Estimation of Gastrin (A), C-reactive protein (B) in experimental animals. Values were expressed in Mean ± SEM; n = 8 animals/group. Statistical analysis was performed using two-way ANOVA followed by Bonferroni multiple comparison test, ##, ### indicates P value ≤ 0.01 and 0.001 respectively vs Normal Control Group, *, ** and *** indicates P value ≤ 0.05, 0.01 and 0.001 respectively vs Cancer Control (CC) Group.

substances are linked to cancer progression (Barrera 2012). An increased lipid peroxidation level (p ≤ 0.05) in gastric and liver tissues of cancer control group was observed which concludes involvement of oxidative stress in MNU-induced gastric cancer after 16- and 24 weeks (Fig 4.6(A), (C)). Several evidences report that garlic as well as ginger possess anti-carcinogenic, anti-mutagenic and immune-modulating properties (Chen 1992, Peng, Tao et al. 2012). Antioxidant defense mechanism is considered to mitigate cancerous lesions by scavenging reactive radical species, leading to reduced level of DNA damage mediated by free radicals. A significant reduction in LPO levels in the stomach and liver tissues of both the combination treatment group could be attributed to the intake of bioactive nutrients present in ginger and garlic that are believed to act as scavengers of superoxide anions and hydroxyl radicals (Rice-Evans, Miller et al. 1996, Pérez-Severiano, Rodríguez-Pérez et al. 2004). But the prophylactic combination group was shown to have a significant (p ≤ 0.01) decreased level of LPO in comparison to therapeutic group in both 16 weeks and 24 weeks.

Vast evidences report that ginger and garlic possess anti-carcinogenic, anti-mutagenic and immune-modulating properties (Srinivasan 2017). In this study, it is noted that both the stomach and liver tissues of MNU-induced cancer control group exhibited a significant (p ≤ 0.05) increased antioxidant activity (FRAP) whereas normal rats reduced this parameter. Although there is improvement of antioxidant activity as evidenced by FRAP levels in the stomach and liver tissues of combination effect of garlic and ginger group (Prophylactic and Therapeutic dose) but it is not impressive as that of individual ginger extract, garlic extract and 5-FU treated rats comparable to cancer control rats (Fig 4.6(B), (D)).

## Fig 4.6 Effect of Test Drugs on Some Major Oxidative Stress Markers

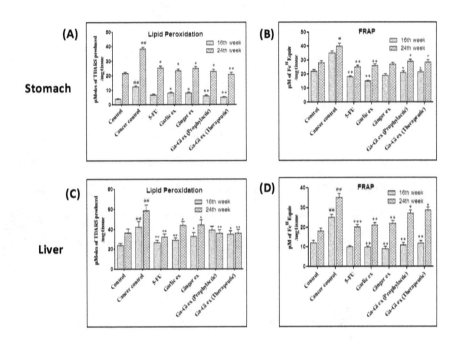

Lipid peroxidation (A), Ferric Reducing Antioxidant Potential (B) in the stomach tissue and Lipid peroxidation (C) and Ferric Reducing Antioxidant Potential (D) on liver tissue of experimental animals. Results are expressed in Mean ± SEM, n = 8 animals/group. Statistical analysis was performed by using two-way Analysis of Variance (ANOVA) using graph pad prism software followed by Bonferroni multiple comparison test. # indicates p value ≤ 0.05, ## indicates p value ≤ 0.01 vs normal rat, *, ** and *** indicates p value ≤ 0.05, 0.01 and 0.001 respectively vs cancer control rat.

### 4.3.3.2 Effect of Test Drugs on Enzymatic Antioxidants

Oxidative stress has been implicated in the development and progression of a variety of metabolic disorders, inflammatory disorders and to many more. Oxidative stress linked with the initiation, promotion, and progression of cancer occurs because of an imbalance between free radical production and antioxidant defenses. Free radical formation occurs continuously in the cells as an outcome of both enzymatic and non-enzymatic reactions involved in the respiratory chain, in phagocytosis, and in the cytochrome P-450 system (Liu, Stern et al. 1999, Lobo, Patil et al. 2010). Enzymatic antioxidants such as Catalase, Superoxide Dismutase (SOD), Glutathione Peroxidase (GPx), Glutathione S-Transferase (GST) are labeled as first line of defense against noxious free radicals like superoxide and hydrogen peroxides which may have deleterious effect on lipid, DNA and protein structure leading to tissue damage (Talas, Ozdemir et al. 2009). As liver is considered to be the major detoxification organ, so a decrease in the activity of these enzymes in liver confirms the diseased status (Ekambaram, Rajendran et al. 2008). So, in our study we checked both the therapeutic and prophylactic efficacy of the drugs on the antioxidant status of MNU-induced gastric cancer in both stomach as well as liver tissues on 16 weeks and 24 weeks of drug treated rats.

Several reports have cited decreased activities of SOD in various carcinogenic conditions (Yang, Chen et al. 2012). The results in this present study corroborate with previous findings that there is a significant ($p \leq 0.01$) decrease in the SOD activity in the stomach and liver tissues of MNU-induced gastric cancer rats. However, an increase in the activity of SOD was observed in the 5-FU, ginger and garlic extract treated group as compared to MNU-induced rats in the stomach and liver tissues of 24 weeks' treatment individually. It is also impressive to report that a significant increase in SOD activity in both the liver and stomach tissues of combination group of garlic and ginger extract has been seen when compared to cancer control rats of 24 weeks of treatment. The observed decline in SOD levels in MNU-induced rats in this study might be because of the increase in circulating lipid peroxides, which reportedly results in the accumulation of superoxide anions that are capable of traversing membranes causing deleterious effects at sites beyond the tumor. Several studies have also reported the decreased expression of SOD is associated with increased incidences of esophageal adenocarcinoma, lung cancer and head and neck squamous cell carcinoma in comparison to normal tissues (Manju and Nalini 2005, Salzman, Kankova et al. 2007, Teoh-Fitzgerald, Fitzgerald et al. 2012). The noticeable decreased SOD activity in the present study in the liver tissue of MNU-induced animals may be attributed to enhanced superoxide radical production during MNU metabolism in the liver of cancer control animals. Evidences from a recent clinical study reported the elevation in SOD level by administering ginger extract as a daily supplement in breast cancer patients (Danwilai, Konmun et al. 2017). In addition to this, another study reported the hepatoprotective effect of ethanolic extract of ginger against acetaminophen-induced acute toxicity was due to the elevation in major antioxidant enzyme SOD (Ajith, Hema et al. 2007). Studies demonstrated the antioxidant and immunomodulative effects of aged black garlic extract was due to the enhanced SOD activity against gastric cancer induced Kunming mice (Wang, Jiao et al. 2012). However, this present investigation gave a new insight in the amelioration of gastric cancer which confirmed the elevated SOD activity of garlic and ginger in combination might be due to protection from superoxide, peroxyl radicals and hydroxyl radicals in a therapeutic and prophylactic manner.

Catalase is widely distributed in all tissues and catalyzes the breakdown of $H_2O_2$ in to water where the source of $H_2O_2$ is the neutralization of superoxide anion ($O^{2-}$) mediated by SOD

(McCord and Fridovich 1969). Catalase which has a significant role against the deleterious effects of lipid peroxidation acts as a preventive endogenous antioxidant. Most of the cancerous condition has shown a decreased level of catalase activity (Thirunavukkarasu and Sakthisekaran 2001). This study revealed a significant ($p \leq 0.01$) decline in catalase activity in both the liver and stomach tissues of MNU-induced rats when compared to normal control rats for 16 weeks as well as 24 weeks of study period. A significant ($p \leq 0.01$) increased level of catalase activity was seen in both the liver and stomach tissues of ginger and garlic individually treated groups and the combination group for 16 and 24 weeks as compared to MNU-induced cancerous rats. This combination treatment group confirms its antioxidant properties due to the presence of various bioactive phytocompounds in garlic and ginger and proved that oxidative injury has been ameliorated in gastric cancer animals. Enhanced catalase activity on combined supplementation of ginger and garlic relative to MNU-induced rats may be due to its free radical scavenging activity and subsequently decreased utilization of antioxidant enzymes. These results justify the marked prophylactic and therapeutic efficacy of ginger garlic combination against MNU-induced gastric cancer. Reports from previous study described the role of ginger extract in increasing the level of catalase in liver cancer (Norliza Ahmad *et al.*, 2006). Likewise, aged garlic extract also displayed significant elevated level in catalase activity against cisplatin induced oxidative injury (Nasr 2014). The elevated catalase activity in this study was substantiated by the above reports which mitigated the oxidative stress by the ginger garlic combination.

GST belongs to a complex supergene-encoded family of detoxification enzymes found in almost all animal tissues (Hayes, Kerr et al. 1989). Like other antioxidant enzymes, a significant decreased activity of GST has been observed in the stomach ($p \leq 0.05$) and liver (p

≤ 0.01) tissues of MNU-induced rats compared to normal control rats in both 16 and 24 weeks. The deficiency of enzymatic antioxidants GST in the blood of cancer control animals may be due to increased utilization of scavenging lipid peroxides as well as sequestration by tumor cells and also due to the decreased availability of GSH (Arivazhagan, Balasenthil et al. 2000). The reduction in the activity of GST is mainly attributable to the liver toxicity caused by the metabolism of MNU which is clearly reflected in the current study. However, the GST activity has reached a substantial increased level in stomach tissue of individual ginger and garlic treated group in 16 weeks and 24 weeks. It is interesting to note that the combination group (prophylactic and therapeutic) in stomach tissue showed a noticeable ($p \leq 0.05$) increased GST activity for 16 and 24 weeks. Analogously in the liver tissues all the test drug treated groups (the individual garlic, ginger extract and combination) have shown a significant ($p \leq 0.01$) increased GST activity for 16 and 24 weeks of drug supplementation. Reports from various studies demonstrated the enhanced detoxification and chemotherapeutic potential of organosulphur compounds of garlic is due to the enhanced GST activity in benzo [a] pyrene–induced neoplasia (Sparnins, Barany et al. 1988). Phytocompounds from ginger have shown to exhibit antitumorigenic effect in chemically induced liver cancer by elevating the level of GST (Taha, Abdul et al. 2010). Results of the present study are also congruent with the above reports which substantiate the elevation of GST is due to the administration of these spices of natural origin.

GPx and GR are predominantly involved in the detoxification of carcinogens, free radicals and peroxides by conjugating the toxic substances with GSH, ultimately protecting the cells against carcinogen-induced cytotoxicity (Klaunig and Kamendulis 2004). Herein, normal rats displayed normal activity of the antioxidant enzyme GPx whereas profound decrease in

GPx activity was observed in the stomach and liver tissues of cancerous animals in 16 weeks and 24 weeks. Depleted level of total sulfyhydryl (TSH) contents or depletion of glutathione may be associated with this antioxidant defense inhibition (Yu 1994). The individual ginger, garlic and 5-FU treated animals in the present investigation showed a significant ($p \leq 0.05$) increased activity whereas co-treatment with ginger and garlic extract showed substantial enhancement ($p \leq 0.01$) in GPx activity which has a better effect on the depleted GPx activity in 16 weeks and 24 weeks of drug treatment both prophylactically and therapeutically. Reports from a clinical study described that the supplementation ginger rhizome powder in early-stage breast cancer patients showed an increase in GPx activity (Karimi and Roshan 2013). Likewise, supplementation of garlic powder diets was found to elevate GPx activity in diethylnitrosamine-induced rat hepatocarcinogenesis (Kweon, Park et al. 2003). Hence, it can be concluded that GPx might be operative to increase its activity which is evident from the elevated level of lipid peroxidation in the present study. Low levels of tissue antioxidant enzymes are likely to result in high levels of tissue damage that are reflected as lipid peroxides, protein carbonyls, etc. (Kota, Krishna et al. 2008). Conversely elevated levels of this antioxidant enzyme mitigated this oxidative damage to tissues which has been observed in this study in terms of decreased lipid peroxides with co-treatment of ginger and garlic.

Analogously, a profound reduction ($p \leq 0.01$) in the level of GR in MNU-induced rats was also noticed in both the liver and stomach tissues compared to normal control rats. Although the treatment with ginger and garlic extract individually elevated ($p \leq 0.01$) the GR level compared to 5-FU group, the combination group exhibited relatively enhanced Glutathione Reductase level ($p \leq 0.01$) in liver and stomach ($p \leq 0.001$) in comparison to the cancer control rats in both 16 weeks and 24 weeks of treatment by prophylactically and therapeutically.

Reports from previous study elicited the enhanced glutathione reductase activity by the garlic oil and its organosulfur compounds in rats fed with high fat diets (Sheen, Chen et al. 1999). Another study described the concomitant dietary feeding of ginger (1%w/w) significantly mitigated lindane-induced lipid peroxidation by subsequent upsurge in the GSH-dependent enzymes glutathione peroxidase and glutathione reductase (Ahmed, Suke et al. 2008). Low levels of GSH and declined activities of GSH-dependent enzymes observed in the MNU-treated rats may be due to the tissue response to oxidative stress during carcinogenesis. Reduced levels of these antioxidants may be due to the over utilization of GSH and its dependent enzymes to scavenge the products of LPO as well as sequestration by tumor cells. The changes in the activities of SOD, Catalase, GST, GPX and GR in the stomach are depicted in Table 4(a) and Table 4(b).

Liver and stomach possess a variety of redox systems comprising the glutathione/glutathione disulfide (GSH/GSSG), cysteine/cystine (Cys/CySS) and reduced and oxidized thioredoxin (Trx/TrxSS), therefore it was worthwhile to investigate the activities of GPx, GR, GST, and SOD in liver and stomach together since they may efficiently scavenge toxic free radicals and be partly responsible for protection against lipid peroxidation due to carcinogen toxicity. Oral administration of the combined treatment of ginger and garlic (100 mg/kg) was found to display a significant attenuation of these antioxidant enzymes in stomach as well as liver. The results obtained in the present investigation conclude that a significant decrease in the activities of SOD, CAT, GR, GPx and GST in both the liver and stomach tissues reveal the relation of oxidative stress and cancerous lesions in MNU-induced rats when compared to normal control rats. Although the individual extract of ginger and garlic significantly increased the activities of these enzymes as compared to MNU-induced rats, the

Table 4(a) Effect of Test Drugs on SOD, Catalase, GST, GPX and GR Level in Stomach Tissue

| Treatment | Enzymatic Oxidative Stress Markers in Stomach | | | | | | | | | |
|---|---|---|---|---|---|---|---|---|---|---|
| | SOD (Unit/min/mg protein) | | CATALASE (nM/min/mg protein) | | GST (nM/min/mg Protein) | | GPx (nM/min/mg Protein) | | GR (nM/min/mg Protein) | |
| | 16th Week | 24th Week | 16th Week | 24th Week | 16th Week | 24th Week | 16th Week | 24th Week | 16th Week | 24th Week |
| Normal Control | 31.06±2.61 | 30.9±2.09 | 30.26±1.50 | 42.60±1.37 | 5.9±0.35 | 10.45±0.67 | 16.26±0.96 | 20.56±1.98 | 16.44±1.90 | 25.56±2.50 |
| Cancer Control | 16.94±1.02## | 17.08±1.98## | 12.94±1.71### | 26.80±1.65## | 2.9±0.29## | 6.9±0.45## | 7.0±0.78## | 14.0±192## | 10.53±1.10## | 16.67±1.79## |
| 5-FU | 21.2±1.27** | 21.56±1.32** | 17.07±1.98** | 32.80±1.16** | 3.95±0.18* | 7.89±0.56 | 10.58±0.90* | 15.95±1.95 | 12.45±1.50* | 19.08±1.09** |
| Garlic extract | 19.8±1.24* | 23.7±1.32** | 16.78±1.89 | 29.98±1.98* | 5.67±0.56** | 8.89±0.65** | 8.42±0.25 | 16.98±1.38* | 12.89±1.43* | 20.98±1.86** |
| Ginger extract | 18.9±1.26* | 24.50±1.34** | 17.87±1.98* | 29.90±1.87* | 4.34±0.29* | 7.9±0.61 | 9.87±1.02 | 15.67±1.46 | 11.91±0.79 | 20.09±1.87 |
| Garlic-Ginger extract (Prophylactic dose) | 21.64±1.35** | 22.67±1.16** | 24.98±1.2** | 34.0±1.41*** | 5.89±0.56** | 9.08±0.69** | 14.89±1.09** | 16.78±1.45* | 14.87±1.67** | 24.67±1.98*** |
| Garlic-Ginger extract (Therapeutic dose) | 24.98±1.38*** | 26.0±1.56*** | 26.87±1.9*** | 36.9±1.91*** | 6.89±0.34** | 8.99±0.87 | 14.85±1.23** | 17.8±1.43** | 15.78±1.87** | 26.87±2.10*** |

Results are expressed in Mean ± SEM, n = 6 animals/group. Statistical analysis was performed by using two-way Analysis of Variance (ANOVA) using graph pad prism software followed by Bonferroni multiple comparison test. # indicates p value ≤ 0.05, ## indicates p value ≤ 0.01 vs normal rat, *, ** and *** indicates p value ≤ 0.05, ≤ 0.01 and ≤ 0.001 respectively vs cancer control rat.

**Table 4(b) Effect of Test Drugs on SOD, Catalase, GST, GPX and GR Level in Liver Tissue**

| Treatment | Enzymatic Oxidative Stress Markers in Liver ||||||||||
|---|---|---|---|---|---|---|---|---|---|---|
| | SOD (Unit/min/mg protein) || CATALASE (nM/min/mg protein) || GST (nM/min/mg Protein) || GPx (nM/min/mg Protein) || GR (nM/min/mg Protein) ||
| | 16th Week | 24th Week | 16th Week | 24th Week | 16th Week | 24th Week | 16th Week | 24th Week | 16th Week | 24th Week |
| Normal Control | 21.06±2.61 | 35.09±2.09 | 35.26±1.94 | 45.60±1.99 | 15.09±0.55 | 20.45±0.97 | 13.26±0.90 | 20.56±1.98 | 18.44±1.90 | 35.56±2.50 |
| Cancer Control | 10.94±1.02$^{\#\#}$ | 24.08±1.98$^{\#\#}$ | 22.94±1.71$^{\#\#}$ | 25.80±1.65$^{\#\#\#\#}$ | 7.90±0.29$^{\#\#}$ | 13.90±0.45$^{\#\#}$ | 8.90±0.78$^{\#\#}$ | 12.0±1.78$^{\#\#}$ | 10.53±1.10$^{\#\#}$ | 25.67±1.79$^{\#\#}$ |
| 5-FU | 13.20±1.27$^{*}$ | 26.56±1.32$^{*}$ | 15.07±1.18 | 30.80±1.86$^{*}$ | 9.95±0.28$^{**}$ | 14.89±0.56 | 9.58±0.99$^{*}$ | 14.95±0.95$^{*}$ | 13.45±1.50$^{*}$ | 27.08±1.89$^{*}$ |
| Garlic extract | 12.80±1.24 | 25.70±1.32 | 16.78±1.29 | 31.98±1.98$^{**}$ | 8.67±0.56 | 15.89±0.65$^{*}$ | 8.42±0.25 | 16.98±1.38$^{*}$ | 11.89±1.43 | 28.98±1.86$^{*}$ |
| Ginger extract | 12.90±1.26 | 29.50±1.34$^{**}$ | 19.87±1.38$^{*}$ | 29.90±1.87$^{**}$ | 8.34±0.29 | 15.90±0.61 | 9.87±1.02$^{*}$ | 15.67±1.46 | 11.91±1.39 | 28.09±1.80$^{*}$ |
| Garlic-Ginger extract (Prophylactic dose) | 18.64±1.35$^{***}$ | 33.67±1.16$^{***}$ | 30.98±1.80$^{**}$ | 38.0±1.91$^{***}$ | 10.89±0.56$^{**}$ | 16.08±0.69 | 10.89±1.09 | 16.78±1.45 | 15.87±1.67$^{**}$ | 29.67±1.98$^{**}$ |
| Garlic-Ginger extract (Therapeutic dose) | 19.98±1.38$^{***}$ | 34.0±1.56$^{***}$ | 31.87±1.90$^{**}$ | 39.90±1.92$^{***}$ | 11.89±0.44$^{**}$ | 18.99±0.87 | 11.85±1.23$^{**}$ | 18.80±1.43$^{**}$ | 16.78±1.68$^{**}$ | 32.87±2.10$^{***}$ |

Results are expressed in Mean ± SEM, n = 6 animals/group. Statistical analysis was performed by using two-way Analysis of Variance (ANOVA) using graph pad prism software followed by Bonferroni multiple comparison test. $^{\#}$ indicates p value ≤ 0.05, $^{\#\#}$ indicates p value ≤ 0.01 vs normal rat, $^{*}$, $^{**}$ and $^{***}$ indicates p value ≤ 0.05, ≤ 0.01 and ≤ 0.001 respectively vs cancer control rat.

combination groups have shown to normalize the values of these enzymes in a more promising manner both in the stomach and liver tissues in 16 weeks and 24 weeks of drug administration both prophylactically and therapeutically. Thus, both ginger and garlic extract classified as functional foods based on their ability to ameliorate oxidative stress induced by carcinogenesis.

### 4.3.3.3 Effect of Test Drugs on Nonenzymatic Antioxidants

Numerous evidences exist on the significant contribution of free radicals towards the progression of cancer and its complications. Enzymatic free radical species denotes a variety of highly reactive molecules which includes reactive oxygen intermediates (ROI) like O-, OH-,ROO, reactive nitrogen species (RNS) like nitric oxide (Halliwell 1995, Sen 2001). Excess production of these free radicals in response to the cellular oxidative stress is lethal to cell growth, intercellular signaling regulation and immune system. Endogenous anti-oxidant system promotes detoxification which includes a number of enzymatic antioxidants and non-enzymatic anti-oxidants. Reduced glutathione (GSH) and vitamin C and vitamin E are the major non-enzymatic antioxidants which act as a second line of defense mechanism that scavenge the active radicals to suppress chain initiation. These antioxidants were found to delay or inhibit cellular damage mainly through their free radical scavenging property (Halliwell 1995). A decrease in these antioxidant capacities has been observed in cancer patients by several research groups (Poprac, Jomova et al. 2017).

Reduced glutathione is an important non-protein thiol of redox cycle in conjugation with GPx and GST protects cells against chemical carcinogenesis by scavenging ROS (Navarro, Obrador et al. 1997). So changes in the dynamics of cancer cell proliferation are accompanied by changes in their redox status that consequently could be reflected in their antioxidant machinery (Hall 1999, Navarro, Obrador et al. 1999). This non-enzymatic antioxidant enzyme serves as inhibitors at initiation and transformation stages of carcinogenesis and can ultimately act as anti-carcinogens. Depletion of GSH occurs because of prolonged oxidative challenge. Substantiating to this mechanism, a significant reduction in the level of GSH in the stomach ($p \leq 0.05$) and liver ($p \leq 0.01$) tissues of cancer control rats was noticed compared to normal control rats in both 16 weeks and 24 weeks while the individual garlic extract and ginger extract treatment groups has tried to increase the GSH level in both stomach and liver tissues compared to MNU-induced rats and is shown in (Fig 4.7(A), (C)). Surprisingly, the combination dose of garlic and ginger extract group has shown a significantly increased level of reduced glutathione in both stomach and liver tissue of 16 and 24 weeks both prophylactically and therapeutically. Consistent with the above report, decreased GSH level in MNU-induced rats occurred owing to the increased utilization for scavenging free radicals along with detoxification of MNU. The administration of the combination dose of ginger and garlic extract increased the GSH level to near normal levels probably by modulating oxidative stress. An *in vivo* study reported the use of ginger administration elevated the level of reduced glutathione in diabetic rats (Shanmugam, Mallikarjuna et al. 2011). Another study elicited the concomitant dietary feeding of ginger also significantly increased the reduced glutathione level in malathion induced oxidative stress in albino Wistar rats (Ahmed, Seth et al. 2000). Evidences also reported that administration of organosulphur compounds in garlic elevated the levels of intracellular GSH in liver carcinoma (Chen, Pung et al. 2004). The results of the present study are also in line with the previous reports on the activity of ginger and garlic in ameliorating oxidative stress by elevating the reduced glutathione level.

Antioxidants like vitamin C and E exhibit many biological functions such as free radical scavenging, immune stimulation and activation of carcinogen (van Poppel and van den Berg

1997). Vitamin C which is an extracellular antioxidant restrains the host resistance against cancer development, initiation and progression. The major function of vitamin C is the restoration of cellular integrity of cell membrane from oxidative damage through neutralization of free radicals and regeneration of antioxidants from vitamin E and also to prevent the GSH from oxidation (Beyer 1994). The current study revealed a significant decreased ($p \leq 0.01$) level of vitamin C in the stomach tissue and a noticeable decrease ($p \leq 0.05$) in liver tissue of MNU-induced cancer animals in comparison to normal rats. Notably, garlic extract, ginger extract and their combination significantly increased ($p \leq 0.01$) the level of this non-enzymatic antioxidant in both liver and stomach tissues as compared with cancer control animals (Fig 4.7(B), (D)). Therefore, the decreased concentrations of vitamin C and GSH in MNU-induced rats may be due to the increased utilization of these antioxidants to neutralize the TBARS level while the combination of ginger and garlic retained the near normal level of these non-enzymatic antioxidants in MNU-induced rats. This might be because of the potent free radical scavenging and antioxidant properties of ginger and garlic by which these two spices also noted to help in eliminating DNA-carcinogen interaction, hence avoids carcinogenesis. Vitamin C may affect carcinogenesis by blocking the formation of nitrosanimes, antioxidant effects and acceleration of detoxification of liver enzymes (Glatthaar, Hornig et al. 1986, Lobo, Patil et al. 2010). The upregulation of vitamin C by the combined treatment of ginger and garlic in the present study to mitigate the pathophysiology of carcinogenesis was probably due to the antioxidant effects of the natural phytoconstituents present in them which was also obtained in the *in vitro* studies on the phytocompounds such as [6]-Gingerol, alliin and the whole extracts of ginger and garlic in our study. Previous studies also described the garlic organosulfur compounds reported to

**Fig 4.7 Effect of Test Drugs on Some Major Non-Enzymatic Antioxidants**

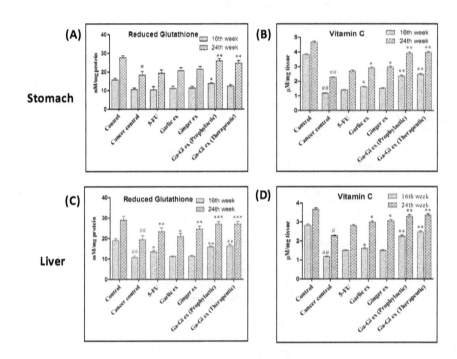

Reduced Glutathione (A), Vitamin C (B) in the stomach tissue and Reduced Glutathione (C) and Vitamin C (D) on liver tissue of experimental animals. Results are expressed in Mean ± SEM, n = 8 animals/group. Statistical analysis was performed by using two-way Analysis of Variance (ANOVA) using graph pad prism software followed by Bonferroni multiple comparison test. # indicates p value ≤ 0.05, ## indicates p value ≤ 0.01 vs normal rat, *, ** and *** indicates p value ≤ 0.05, 0.01 and 0.001 respectively vs cancer control rat.

elevate the vitamin C level in n-nitrosodiethylamine-induced carcinogenesis which helps in scavenging of reactive oxygen species (Sundaresan and Subramanian 2003).

#### 4.3.3.4  Gene Expression of Oxidative Stress Markers

To reveal the mechanism behind the suppression of oxidative stress by our tested drug on MNU-induced carcinogenesis, gene expression study of two major redox proteins namely Thioredoxin (TRx) and Glutaredoxin (GRx) were performed in the stomach tissue of the experimental animals after 24 weeks of drug treatment. TRx and GRx are a class of small redox proteins which maintains cellular redox homeostasis, cell survival and are highly expressed in many cancers which also act as antioxidants by facilitating the reduction of other proteins by cysteine thiol-disulfide exchange. They also exert their antioxidant functions through either directly quenching singlet oxygen and scavenging hydroxyl radicals, or indirectly by reducing oxidized ROS target proteins (Karlenius and Tonissen 2010, Bhatia, McGrath et al. 2016). Reports revealed that higher expression level of thioredoxin in human primary gastric tumors corresponds to higher proliferative and survival rate than tumors that do not express thioredoxin (Grogan, Fenoglio-Prieser et al. 2000). The expression of TRx and GRx are expressed in terms of fold change with respect to the house keeping gene, β-actin. TRx as well as GRx displayed a significantly ($p \leq 0.001$) three-fold increased level in cancer control rats in comparison to normal rats. However, the level of both TRx and GRx was shown to have an apparent ($p \leq 0.01$) two-fold decrease in the ginger, garlic and the combination group (prophylactic and therapeutic dose) in comparison to MNU-induced cancer group which is much better than 5-FU treated animals (Fig 4.8 (A), (B)). Hence, it can be concluded that the two spices mitigate oxidative stress in cancerous conditions by improving endogenous anti-oxidant system mediated by the genes involved in the thiol system.

### 4.3.4 Anti-Inflammatory Potential of Test Drugs

#### 4.3.4.1 Gene Expression of Inflammatory Markers

Nuclear factor-kappaB (NF-kB), the master regulator of inflammation mediates a crosstalk between inflammation and cancer at multiple levels. Upraised NF-κB level in tumorous tissues, create a pro-tumorigenic microenvironment by accumulating several pro-inflammatory cytokines at the tumor site. NF-κB is a transcriptional regulator mediating COX-2 expression which may be related to cell proliferation in human gastric cancer cells (Lim, Kim et al. 2001). Nuclear expression of NF-κB was significantly more frequently observed in gastric cancer tissues than in nonmalignant gastric tissues (Wu, Chen et al. 2007). The NF-κB pathway regulates pro-inflammatory cytokines (TNFα, IL-6, IL-2, IL-10, PGE2) production, leukocyte recruitment, and cell survival which are important contributors to the inflammatory response (Lawrence 2009). During inflammatory responses, the macrophages get activated which release excess amount of various inflammatory mediators such as NO and PGE2 and of pro-inflammatory cytokines such as IL-1β, IL-6, and TNF-α which are responsible for many chronic inflammatory diseases and cancer (Lin and Karin 2007). The present study revealed the effect of ginger and garlic extract and the combination of the two (prophylactic and therapeutic dose) spices on the expression of some pro-inflammatory genes in stomach lesions after 24 weeks of drug treatment to find out how inflammation is mediated in MNU-induced gastric carcinoma. The level of pro-inflammatory markers like IL-6, IL-2, IL-10 and COX-2 has shown a significant fold change in cancer control group in comparison to control animals (Fig 4.9(A), (B), (C), (D)). However, the combined treatment of ginger and garlic has significantly ($p \leq 0.01$) decreased the expression level of IL-2, IL-10 and COX-2 both prophylactically and therapeutically which is comparable to 5-FU group. Reports from various studies also

**Fig 4.8 Modulatory Effect of Test Drugs on Thioredoxin and Glutaredoxin by Gene Expression Studies**

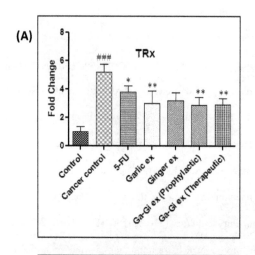

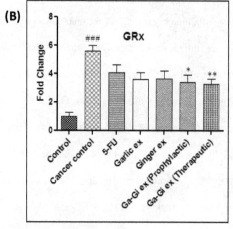

TRx (A) and GRx (B) gene expression in the stomach tissue of experimental animals. Values were expressed in Mean ± SEM; n = 8 animals/group. Statistical analysis was performed using one way ANOVA followed by Tukey's multiple comparison test, ##, ### indicates P value ≤ 0.01 and 0.001 respectively vs Normal Control Group, *, ** and *** indicates P value ≤ 0.05, 0.01 and 0.001 respectively vs Cancer Control (CC) Group.

confirmed the link between high levels of IL-6 and IL-8 and increased risk of lung cancer (Pine, Mechanic et al. 2011). An *in vivo* study with mice treated with broccoli rich in sulforaphane displayed decreased expression of tumor necrosis factor (TNF)-α and IL-1β in the gastric mucosa, contributing to amelioration of inflammation in high salt-induced gastric ulcer (Yanaka, Fahey et al. 2009). The results of the present study obtained corroborate with the above report which suggest that the combination of phytocompounds present in ginger and garlic prevented inflammation in gastric cancer by ameliorating pro-inflammatory cytokines. While in the case of IL-6, although the combination group tried to decrease the expression in a significant manner ($p \leq 0.05$) the ginger extract group alone exhibited a more pronounced decrease ($p \leq 0.01$) which probably may be due to the individual phytoconstituents in ginger. The gene expression of pro-inflammatory cytokines TNF-α, PGE2 in cancer control rats has shown a significant ($p \leq 0.01$) two-fold increase in comparison to normal rats while both the combination group in revealed a two-fold ($p \leq 0.01$) reduced expression of level of TNF-α, PGE2 (Fig 4.10(A), (B), (C)). The expression of NF-κB has shown to reduce significantly ($p \leq 0.001$) by the combination group of ginger and garlic (therapeutic dose) after 24 week of drug treatment. Hence, confirms that the ginger and garlic combination exerted anti-inflammatory activity by inhibiting pro-inflammatory markers like NF-κB, TNFα and IL-6 both prophylactic and therapeutic manner. Reduction of inflammation molecules through the combined effect of ginger and garlic supports that the combination therapeutic effect of ginger and garlic may act as a promising therapeutic agent for the treatment of inflammation-related diseases and gastric cancer. The results of the present investigation were shown to be in line with the *in silico* and *in vitro* study which displayed a promising potential of individual phytocompounds of ginger and garlic in inhibiting NF-κB (Fig 2.1, 2.2) and COX-2 (Fig 3.3).

**Fig 4.9 Modulatory Effect of Test Drugs on Some Major Pro-Inflammatory Markers of Stomach by RT-PCR**

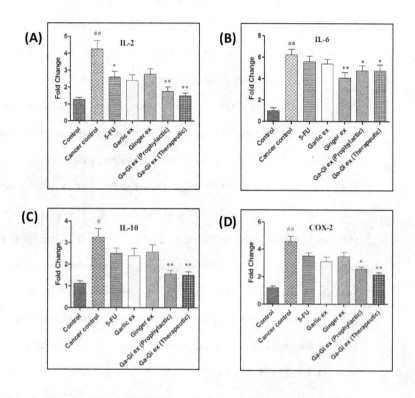

IL-2 (A), IL-6 (B), IL-10 (C) and COX-2 (D) expression in experimental animals. Values were expressed in Mean ± SEM; n = 8 animals/group, statistical analysis was performed using one way ANOVA followed by Tukey's multiple comparison test, ##, ### indicates P value ≤ 0.01 and 0.001 respectively vs Normal Control Group, *, ** and *** indicates P value ≤ 0.05, 0.01 and 0.001 respectively vs Cancer Control (CC) Group.

### 4.3.5 Effect of Test Drugs on Apoptosis

Apoptosis is a major cellular process for the normal development of cell and tissue homeostasis. In this type of suicidal mechanism, cell participates in its own death by an event of caspase activation. Damage of a cell occurs in three different ways, firstly, it will be arrested in the G0 phase where the DNA damage can be repaired before it enters S phase, secondly the cell will undergo necrosis or thirdly it undergoes its natural death which is known as apoptosis. Different types of physiological stimuli such as UV radiation, DNA damage, activation of oncogenes or deprivation of growth factors induce apoptosis (Pervin, Singh et al. 2001). Subsequently, apoptosis results in cell shrinkage, membrane blebbing, chromatin condensation and degradation of DNA into inter-nucleosomal fragments (Elmore 2007).

Apoptosis which ultimately leads to the fragmentation of cell is induced by a complex death program. Two apoptotic signaling pathways exist to induce this death program namely the extrinsic pathway and the intrinsic pathway (Thompson 1995). The extrinsic pathway is initiated by cell death receptors on the cell surface which can be activated by binding to TNF-α or Fas ligand which leads to intracellular apoptotic machinery whereas the intrinsic pathway is mediated by mitochondria and occurs because of DNA damage caused by different chemotherapeutic drugs and radiation. Both pathways activate the key proteolytic caspases. The major key regulator of apoptosis is the Bcl2 protein whose expression modulates the intrinsic apoptotic pathway by controlling the release of cytochrome c from the mitochondria required for activation of caspases (Youle and Strasser 2008). It is known that Bcl2 protein downregulation results in the induction of apoptosis. Fig 4.11(A) represents the immunoblot analysis of pro apoptotic and anti-apoptotic proteins, Bax, Bcl2, Cyt-c, Caspase-9 and Caspase-

**Fig 4.10 Modulatory Effect of Test Drugs on Some Major Pro-Inflammatory Markers of Stomach by RT-PCR**

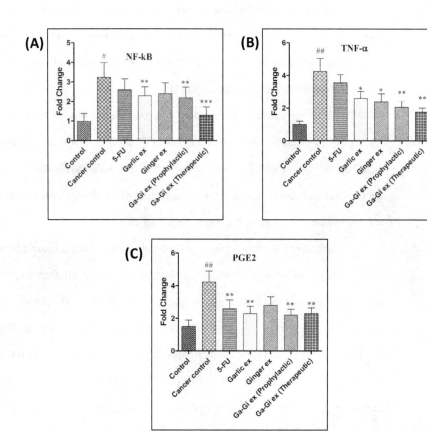

Nf-kB (A), TNF-α (B) and PGE2 (C) expression in experimental animals. Values were expressed in Mean ± SEM; n = 8 animals/group, statistical analysis was performed using one way ANOVA followed by Tukey's multiple comparison test, ##, ### indicates P value ≤ 0.01 and 0.001 respectively vs Normal Control Group, *, ** and *** indicates P value ≤ 0.05, 0.01 and 0.001 respectively vs Cancer Control (CC) Group.

3 in the control and experimental animals. Quantitative data expressing the protein levels were assessed using densitometer and is expressed as fold change (Fig 4.11 (B)-(F)).

The data revealed that there was an upregulated expression of Bcl2 in MNU-alone induced rats, which are in line with the other reports (Ribeiro, Salvadori et al. 2005). In addition to this, another study also reported the apoptotic potential of ginger is associated with downregulation of Bax (Citronberg, Bostick et al. 2013). Some findings also suggested a promising apoptotic potential by garlic-derived sulfur compounds in cancer chemoprevention and chemotherapy (Cerella, Dicato et al. 2011). Supplementation with ginger extract, garlic extract and mostly with the combination of both strongly inhibited Bcl2 protein expression. MNU-induced gastric cancer animals showed a significant increase in the levels of Bcl2 with subsequent decrease in the levels of Bax, Cyt c in comparison to control animals. Treatment with ginger extract, garlic extract and mostly with the combination group (prophylactic and therapeutic dose) showed significant decrease in the level of anti-apoptotic protein Bcl2 with subsequent increase in the levels of proapoptotic proteins Bax and Cyt c.

Caspases belong to a family of proteases which are the central component of the proteolytic system of apoptosis. They play a crucial role to inactivate the proteins that protect living cells from apoptosis. Activation of initiator caspases (Caspase-2,8,9) occur through the apoptotis-signalling which in turn activate the effector caspases (Caspase-3,6,7) to accomplish the major events of apoptosis (Lifshitz, Lamprecht et al. 2001). Ginger extract, garlic extract and the combination group (prophylactic and therapeutic dose) showed significantly increased expression of Caspase-9 and Caspase-3 when compared to MNU-induced group. Low expression level of Caspase-9 and Caspase-3 has been observed in control and MNU-induced group. The prophylactic and therapeutic dose of combination group significantly ($p \leq 0.05$)

**Fig 4.11 Effect of Test Drugs on Apoptotic Proteins by Western Blotting**

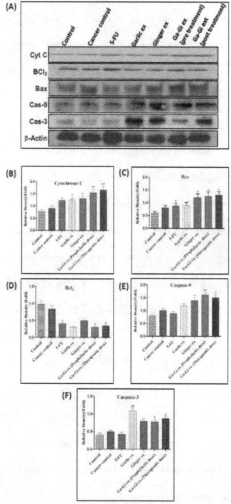

Immunoblotting analysis (A) and bar graphs represent quantification of Cytochrome C (B), Bax (C), Bcl2 (D), Caspase-9 (E), Caspase-3 (F) in control and experimental group of animals. The levels of apoptotic proteins (Cytochrome C, Bax, BCl2, Caspase-9 and Caspase-3) were accordingly plotted as bar charts by keeping β-Actin as a house keeping gene. * ($p \leq 0.05$) and ** ($p \leq 0.01$) in compared to cancer control cells.

increased the proapoptotic proteins Bax, Cyt c, caspase-9 and caspase-3 in comparison to cancer control group which is also comparably high than the individual ginger and garlic extract treated group. The above results are in congruence with the *in vitro* studies on AGS cell lines which attest the apoptotic potential of the major bioactive compound of ginger i.e [6]-Gingerol and Alliin, the major phytocompound of garlic. However, the present *in vivo* study declare that it was not only the presence of [6]-Gingerol and Alliin but also the other bioactive principles of ginger and garlic in combination which are responsible for apoptotic potential of these spices against MNU-induced gastric cancer.

### 4.3.6 Histological Analysis

Histological analysis confirms the pathological changes in the experimental animals and substantiates the influence of the test drugs. Herein in the present study, control animals possessed normal keratinization in the non-glandular epithelium likewise the glandular stomach exhibited normal mucosa and glands whereas the MNU induced cancer rats divulged that the non-glandular stomach epithelium was hypertrophic with vacuolations and orthokeratotic hyperkeratosis and the glandular stomach region exposed areas of mucosal vacuolations, glandular dilatations, focal glandular hyperplasia in $16^{th}$ weeks of MNU induction which was comparatively higher than that of 8 weeks of MNU-induction (Fig 4.12). This affirmed induction of gastric cancer by MNU over a period of 16 weeks. It is interesting to note that the non-glandular stomach epithelium showed orthokeratotic hyperkeratosis while some healing was seen in the glandular stomach as evidenced by occasional vacuolations and degeneration of glands in 5-FU treated rats. After the $16^{th}$ week, it was noticed that in the non-glandular stomach, epithelium and keratinization was normal and in the glandular stomach, except for occasional focal hyperplasia of glands, gastric epithelium appeared normal in both the combination of

**Fig 4.12 Histopathological Changes of Gastric Mucosa in the Experimental Groups**

| Groups | Stomach (10X) 16 weeks | Stomach (10X) 24 weeks |
|---|---|---|
| Control | 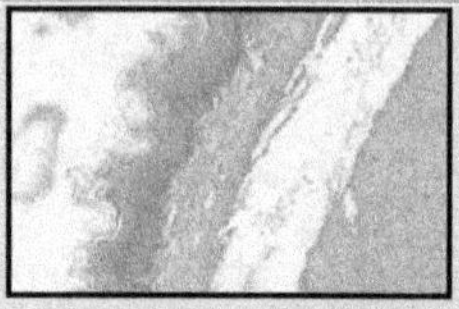 | 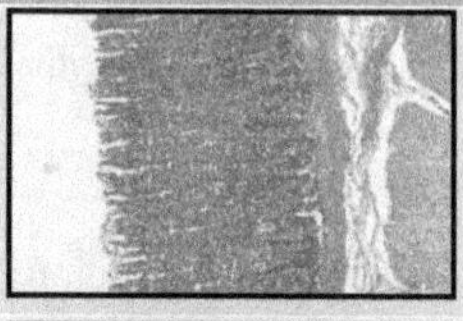 |
| Cancer Control (CC) | 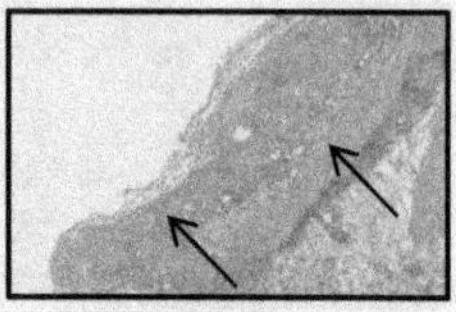 | 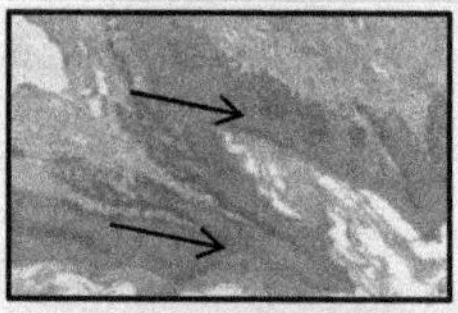 |
| CC + 5-FU | 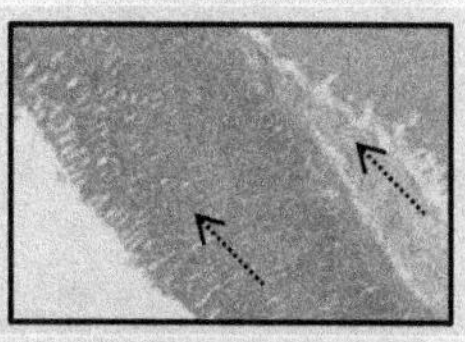 | 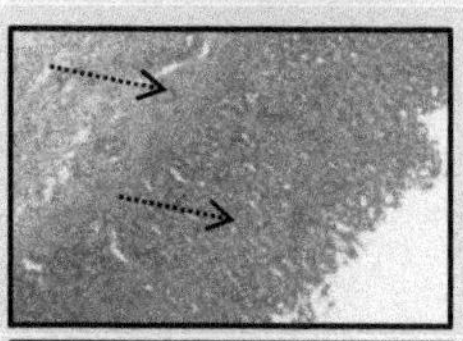 |
| CC + Garlic Extract (Ga) | 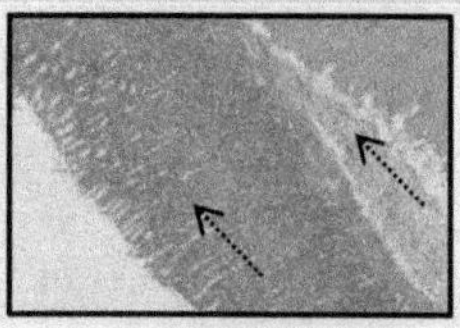 | 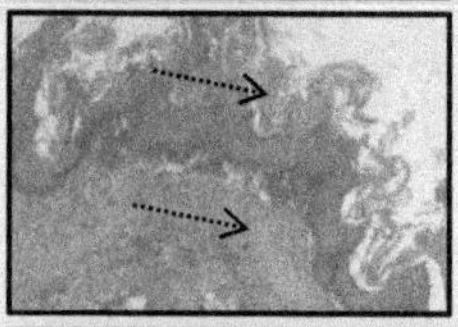 |
| CC + Ginger Extract (Gi) | 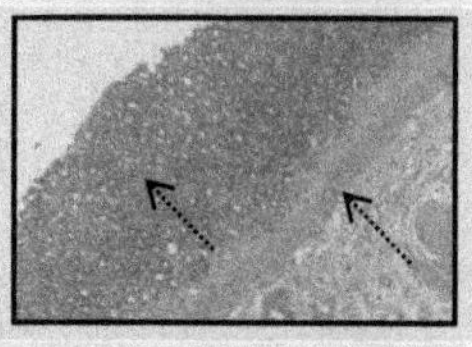 | 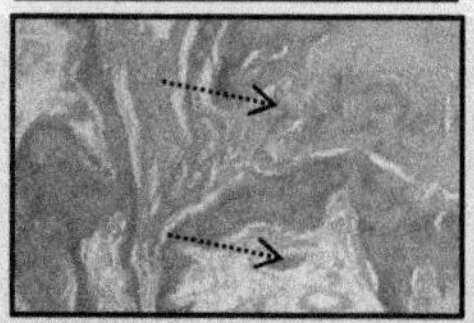 |
| CC + Ga-Gi Extract (Prophylactic Dose) | 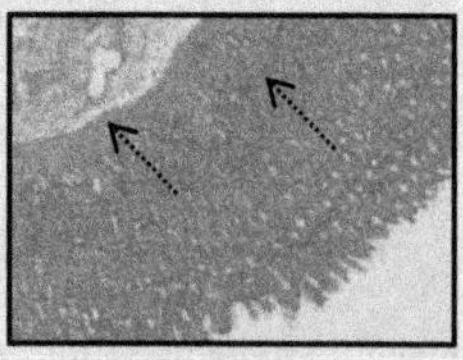 | 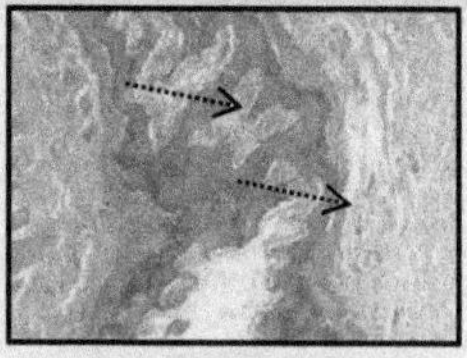 |
| CC + Ga-Gi extract (Therapeutic Dose) | 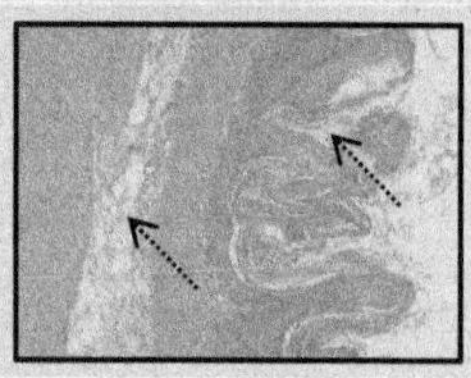 | 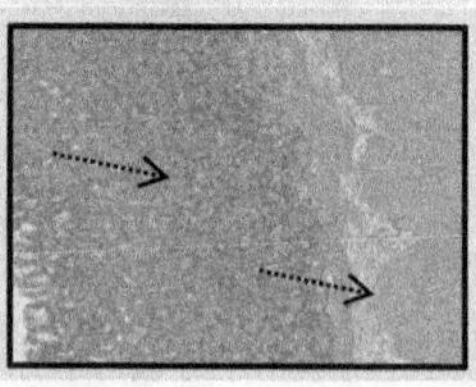 |

Histopathological slides of stomach of different experimental groups stained with Haematoxylin and Eosin. Arrows (↖) in cancer control rats represent the cancerous lesions created by MNU. Arrows (⇢) indicate the lesions in the gastric glands being alleviated by the test drugs.

ginger and garlic extract (therapeutic and prophylactic) treated rats. Although some healing has been observed in the individual treatment groups of ginger and garlic extract but the extent of healing of cancerous lesions observed in prophylactic group was found to be more in comparison to therapeutic group. This clearly confirms the protective role of ginger and garlic in elevating the lesion caused due to experimental induction of gastric cancer and substantiates its chemo preventive action and confirms the synergetic action of both ginger and garlic as identified by *in vitro* studies.

## 4.4 Conclusion

Administration of MNU with 5% NaCl in drinking water to animals for a period of 16 weeks induced gastric cancer which closely mimics the pathologies in humans. Hence, the prophylactic and therapeutic efficacy of ginger and garlic individually and in combination was evaluated in this rodent model which was confirmed by biochemical and molecular tools. The probable mechanism of the anticancer potential of ginger and garlic extract is portrayed in Fig 4.13. Some of the salient features which confirm the tested drugs for its anti-cancer efficiency and its possible mechanism includes as follows.

- The anti-oxidant capacity of ginger and garlic extract individually and in combination in mitigating oxidative stress is significant as noted by the improvement in the endogenous anti-oxidant system
- Co-Treatment with ginger and garlic extract individually and in combination is beneficial in alleviating inflammation associated gastric cancer complications. The combination is more potent as evidenced by suppressed pro-inflammatory markers in the gastric lesions.
- In addition to this, the apoptotic potential of the combination further substantiates the anticancer potential.

**Fig 4.13 Possible Mechanism of Anticancer Potential of Ginger and Garlic Extract in Synergism**

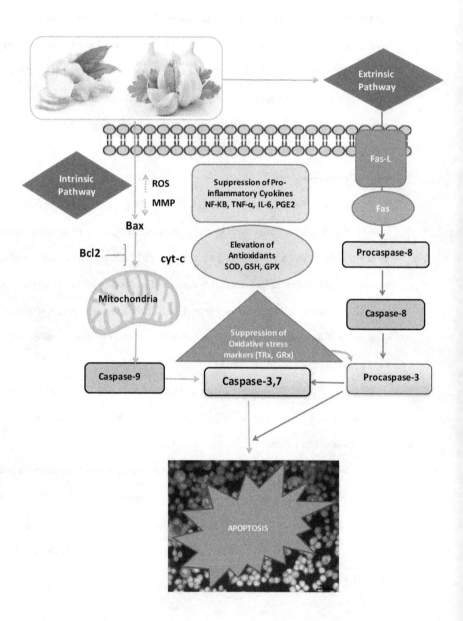

- Dietary intake of ginger and garlic both individually and in combination is worth as this exhibits prophylactic and therapeutic efficacy against inflammation of gastric epithelium leading to gastric ulcers cancer of the stomach.

# CHAPTER 5

## Summary, Conclusion and Recommendation

# CHAPTER 5

## 5.1 Summary

The uncontrolled growth of cancerous cells known as metastasis is a long term multifaceted dynamic process which leads to the development of cancer. Natural products are key agents used for preventing and managing devastating diseases like cancer encountered by mankind. More specifically, they exhibit anticancer potential owing to the existence of bioactive compounds in them such as flavonoids, anthocyanins, lignins, sterols, etc. Likewise, micronutrients in natural product derived diet such as vitamins, trace elements and antioxidants play a pivotal role in reducing cell damage and may act synergistically to enhance several protective mechanisms against carcinogenesis. Researchers have demonstrated that several dietary components of natural origin possess the capacity to prevent and manage cancer. The possible mechanisms include increased detoxification of carcinogens, cell differentiation, maintenance of DNA repair, decrease in cell proliferation and increased apoptosis/autophagy of cancer cells mediated by antioxidant effects and alteration in mitochondrial membrane potential, ER stress etc. Unlike other diseases, cancer exhibits an uncanny ability to remain incognizant to a wide range of treatment approaches. This quality could be attributed to many reasons behind the cause and management of cancer. One such complicated cancer type owing to the various causative agents is gastric cancer affecting more than one million people throughout the world. Further, the identification of the disease at an early stage is farfetched as there are no early diagnostic biomarkers identified for gastric cancer. To add on, treatment of gastric cancer involves a heavy dose of strong drugs which have severe side effects. The repercussions of treatment include early mortality along with organ failure. Hence, identifying functional drugs/foods with fewer side effects which can exhibit both prophylactic and therapeutic effect is worth identifying.

Drug discovery and development through rigorous R&D is a tedious, time and resource driven process. Hence, in the present study two commonly used spices ginger and garlic and its phytoconstituents which also possess medicinal property was selected to reveal its anticancer potential both individually and in combination by *in silico*, *in vitro* and *in vivo* studies.

Computer facilitated approaches such as docking, pharmacophore modelling and virtual screening would potentially save time and resource in drug discovery and development, directing to more promising novel agents and expediting the process. Drug discovery is anticipated to be expedited through the combined use of experimentation and bioinformatics. Inflammation and apoptosis are two major hallmarks of cancer pathology and identifying specific targets to maneuver these pathologies would be ideal to manage the deadly disease. Therefore, to find out the best bioactive lead present in ginger and garlic to combat cancer, the *in-silico* docking analysis of different phytocompounds of ginger ([6]-Gingerol, [10]-Gingerol, [8]-Shogal, Zingerone) and garlic (Alliin, Allicin, Diallydisulphide, *S*-allyl cysteine) with pro-inflammatory markers and apoptotic markers was studied. [6]-Gingerol and Alliin interact strongly with NFkB and COX-2. Likewise, they showed strong binding energy with the apoptotic markers Bax and Bcl2 in comparison to the other molecules of ginger and garlic. Hence, these bioactive leads ([6]-Gingerol and Alliin) were chosen for all *in-vitro* molecular mechanistic studies.

After identifying that the two compounds are potent by *in silico* analysis, [6]-Gingerol, the major phytocompound from Ginger as well as Alliin, the abundant phytoconstituent in Garlic were quantified by HPLC in both fresh and dried forms. It was found out that [6]-

Gingerol content in the aqueous extract of fresh ginger was more in comparison to dried ginger extract. Similarly, Alliin content in the aqueous extract of fresh garlic was observed to be more than the dried garlic extracts. Since cancer pathogenesis involves the generation of many free radicals due to oxidative stress, we found it worth studying the role of these extracts as well as their pure compounds as free radical scavengers by some reliable and reproducible methods which includes 2,2-diphenyl-1-picrylhydrazyl (DPPH), Lipid Peroxidation (LPO) inhibition assay and Ferric reducing antioxidant potential assay (FRAP). These assays confirm the potent antioxidant and free scavenging potential of fresh ginger and garlic extracts in comparison to their dried counterparts.

Subsequently, anticancer efficacy of [6]-Gingerol and Alliin was then assessed using AGS cell lines. Cell viability by MTT assay was performed to check the cytotoxic potential of both [6]-Gingerol and Alliin against AGS cells which showed potent cytotoxic effect at an $IC_{50}$ value of 50 µM (Alliin) and 100 µM ([6]-Gingerol). It is interesting to note that when both compounds were tested against INT-407 normal intestinal cell line, they neither induced proliferation nor inhibited the cell growth. Further to check the morphological features of apoptosis mediated by [6]-Gingerol and Alliin, AO/EB staining was performed which was in accordance with the MTT results and proved that both compounds induced apoptosis. Phosphatidylserine externalization by the Annexin-V assay revealed a higher percentage of early apoptotic cells i.e. 56.4% in the case of Alliin and 37.4% in [6]-Gingerol treated cells by flow cytometric analysis. The percentage of cells actively undergoing early apoptosis as well as late apoptosis by [6]-Gingerol and Alliin showed that these phytocompounds markedly influences apoptosis. Further in order to determine whether suppression of cell proliferation by the test compounds inhibit cell cycle progression, AGS cells treated with $IC_{50}$ dose of both the compounds individually for 24 h was checked for DNA fluorescence in propidium iodide-stained cells by flow cytometer. The results confirmed that [6]-Gingerol caused a buildup of cells in the G2/M phase and cell death in the cancer cells while Alliin caused an inflation of S phase cells and a corresponding reduction of cells in the G2/M phase.

Subsequently to unravel the possible mode of action of the test molecules, AGS cells were monitored by staining with 2, 7-dichlorofluorescein diacetate (DCFH-DA) to identify the presence of ROS. Present investigation confirmed noticeable elevation of intracellular ROS induced by the two phytocompounds ([6]-Gingerol and Alliin) in AGS cells compared to the control cells treated with DMSO. Electron and proton transport through the inner membrane of the mitochondria is liable for cellular ROS generation. Accordingly, the mitochondrial membrane potential is altered by mediating apoptosis. Herein, MMP examined by flow cytometric analysis showed that compared to control, [6]-Gingerol and Alliin individually caused a significant loss of MMP after 24 h of treatment. It was evinced that a loss of MMP may be correlated to the production of ROS in AGS cells upon treatment confirmed by DCFDA staining.

The exact mechanistic pathway in mediating apoptosis of AGS cells induced by Alliin and [6]-Gingerol individually was found worth studying. The results of the immunoblot revealed that the level of Cytochrome c in cytosol was enhanced in AGS cells after treating with Alliin (50 µM and 100 µM) and [6]-Gingerol (100 µM and 250 µM) for 24 h. It suggests that Alliin and [6]-Gingerol improved the level of cytochrome c in cytosol which ultimately activates the caspase-dependent and caspase-independent apoptosis pathway. In this study, activation of caspase-9 and caspase-3 also indicates the unalterable or completing stage of apoptosis. Simultaneously, the level of the anti-apoptotic protein Bcl2 and the proapoptotic protein Bax were determined to characterize the mitochondria mediated apoptosis induced by Alliin and [6]-Gingerol. Immunoblots exhibited downregulation of Bcl2 and the upregulation of Bax. It implied that apoptosis of AGS cells by Alliin and [6]-gingerol was mediated by alteration in the level of Pro and anti-apoptotic proteins of Bcl2 family.

Identifying if there exists any combination effect of the phytoconstituents and the extracts of ginger and garlic was worthful. Hence, in this study we performed drug interaction studies to check existence of different combination effect between [6]-Gingerol and Alliin as well as between individual fresh ginger and fresh garlic extracts. In this context, we found out the existence of a moderate antagonism in between [6]-Gingerol and Alliin. Not surprising aqueous extract of both fresh ginger and fresh garlic exhibited synergetic effect which prompted us to confirm the combined synergetic effect of ginger and garlic extract on MNU-induced gastric cancer in experimental animals.

MNU (100 mg/kg b.w.) in citrate buffer, pH-4.5 along with 5% NaCl induction was standardized in albino Wistar rats via intragastric route initially for a period of 8 weeks and then continued till 16 weeks to check the extent of carcinogenicity in male albino Wistar rats. This chemically induced model mimic's gastric cancer than any other model which was evidenced by the reduction in body weight, water intake as well as feed intake in cancer control animals. Oral treatment of individual garlic and ginger extract as well as the combination of both the extracts were administered to rats to prove the therapeutic efficacy on gastric cancer. The increase in body weight as well as feed intake in drug treated rats is noticeable to prove its efficacy. Gastrin, a specific biomarker of gastric carcinogenesis is elevated in MNU induced gastric cancer rats at two time periods (16 weeks and 24 weeks). However, the significant decrease to 4 folds by ginger, garlic extract and their combination is possibly due to the bioactive ingredients present in it which probably suppress the acute and chronic inflammation caused due to MNU-induced gastric carcinogenesis. Enzymes such as alkaline phosphatase (ALP), Glutamyl transferase (γ-GT) and lactate dehydrogenase (LDH) are considered as diagnostic markers for normal liver functioning. Immunological, metabolic or any other insult to the tissues and organs causes elevation of these enzymes in blood of cancer-induced animals. A significant increase of ALP and LDH activity in serum of cancer induced rats is possibly because of damage of the gastrointestinal tissue. Ginger, garlic extract and their combination treated rats exhibited declined ALP and LDH activity possibly due to the protective effect. The synergetic effect of both the ginger and garlic extract was proved for their prophylactic and therapeutic efficacy. A decrease in γ-GT activity was also observed in serum of cancer control rats which clearly shows that γ-GT is independently associated with risk of cancer specific to the liver and not to stomach cancer.

Oxidative stress associated with increased levels of LPO and other thiobarbituric acid reactive substances are linked to cancer progression. An increased lipid peroxidation level in gastric tissues of cancer control group was observed which confirms involvement of oxidative stress in MNU-induced gastric cancer. A significant reduction in LPO levels of ginger extract, garlic extract and their combination extract administered rats could be due to the intake of bioactive nutrients that are believed to act as scavengers of superoxide anions and hydroxyl radicals. Endogenous antioxidants such as catalase, superoxide dismutase (SOD), glutathione peroxidase (GPx), glutathione S-transferase (GST), glutathione reductase (GR) and reduced glutathione (GSH) are labeled as first line defense against noxious free radicals like superoxide and hydrogen peroxides in cellular tissues. The present study showed a significant reduction in SOD, catalase, GST, GPx and GR activity in both stomach and liver tissue of cancer control rats which may be due to enhanced utilization for scavenging lipid peroxides as well as sequestration by tumor cells. It is interesting to note that ginger extract, garlic extract and their combination treated rats elevated the GST, GPx and GR activity in gastric cancer induced rats which proved the prophylactic and therapeutic efficacy of ginger and garlic extract. Reduced glutathione is an important non-protein thiol which belongs to redox cycle and in conjugation with GPx and GST protects cells against cytotoxicity. So, changes in the dynamics of cancer cell proliferation are accompanied by changes in their intracellular GSH levels that consequently could be reflected in their antioxidant machinery. The present study reported a significant declined level of GSH in cancer control rats compared to normal control rats while the co-treatment of ginger and garlic extract showed an elevated GSH level compared to cancer control rats. The significant elevated expression of Thioredoxins (Trx) and Glutaredoxin (GRx), the key oxidative stress markers in cancer group was due to the increased utilization of these genes for the survival of cancer cells. However, there was a drastic downregulation of TRx, GRx expression in the combined group of ginger and garlic extract in comparison to the cancer group both prophylactically and therapeutically.

The function of inflammation is to eliminate the initial cause of cell injury, clear out the damaged tissues from the inflammatory process, and to initiate tissue repair. During inflammatory responses, the macrophages get activated which release excess amount of various inflammatory mediators such as NO and PGE2 and of pro-inflammatory cytokines such as IL-1ß, IL-6, and TNF-α which are responsible for many chronic inflammatory diseases and cancer. NF-kB is a promoter of inflammatory activities in the body which also regulate proinflammatory genes including IL-1ß, IL-6, and TNF-α. Expression of NF-kB along with the pro-inflammatory markers such as TNF-α, IL-6, IL-10, PGE2 and COX2 revealed a significant upregulation of all the pro-inflammatory markers in cancer group. However, the levels of these pro-inflammatory markers were markedly decreased in the combined group of ginger and garlic extract in comparison to cancer group both prophylactically and therapeutically.

To verify the role of intrinsic and extrinsic pathway involved in the apoptosis, we analyzed the level of Cytochrome c and caspase-9 in the stomach tissue homogenate of experimental animals after 24 weeks of drug treatment. The results infer that ginger and garlic extract in combination significantly improved the level of cytochrome c in cytosol which ultimately activates the caspase-dependent and caspase-independent apoptosis pathway. Simultaneously the level of the anti-apoptotic protein Bcl2 and the proapoptotic protein Bax were determined to characterize the mitochondria mediated apoptosis. Results from this study displayed that apoptosis was mediated by alteration in the level of proapoptotic and anti-apoptotic proteins of Bcl2 family.

Histological analysis confirms the pathological changes in the experimental animals and substantiates the influence of the test drugs. MNU induced cancer control rats divulged non-glandular stomach epithelium which was hypertrophic with vacuolations with focal and atypical glandular hyperplasia. Interestingly, it was noticed that in the non-glandular stomach, epithelium and keratinization was normal in ginger, garlic combination treated rats in comparison to standard drug as well as the individual garlic and ginger treatment group. This clearly confirms the prophylactic and therapeutic protective role of natural foods in elevating the lesion caused due to experimental induction of gastric cancer.

## 5.2 Conclusion

Based on the above study, the prophylactic and therapeutic influence of ginger and garlic extracts together synergistically suppresses the gastric cancer in MNU-induced Albino Wistar rats in a significant manner. The combination of ginger and garlic extract is a potential therapeutic agent to suppress MNU-induced gastric cancer in experimental rats. The probable mode of action of the ginger and garlic extracts in synergism provides a new insight into the chemotherapeutic properties of ginger and garlic, which will allow the design of better management plans for gastric cancer patients. Henceforth, usage of whole extract will be beneficial for the treatment of cancer and its complications rather than its active compounds. The research interest based on ginger and garlic components may provide an approach to decrease the incidence and mortality of gastric cancer. Even though, the free radical scavenging property of *Zingiber officinale and Allium sativum* and its active compounds is found to be almost similar, the anti-oxidant free radical scavenging, anti-inflammatory properties and apoptotic potential shown by the combination dose of *Zingiber officinale and Allium sativum* is found to be superior which will be beneficial in mitigating the several cancer-related complications which are assumed to be majorly caused by oxidative stress. Other than [6]-Gingerol and Alliin, *Zingiber officinale and Allium sativum* contain numerous compounds mediating several biological activities which may synergistically act and may be responsible for its anticancer property. But, the usage of whole extract will be beneficial for the treatment of cancer and its complications rather than its bioactive compounds which will prevent cancer.

## 5.3 Recommendation

This study forms a scientific evidence for the medicinal use of ginger and garlic as anti-cancerous agent and supports its traditional claim by declaring a positive input for a bench to bedside translational research in cancer. Although the results are interesting, further studies are warranted to identify the other mechanisms in mitigating experimentally induced gastric cancers. Subsequently, this could be translated as an adjunct therapy for patients undergoing chemo-radiation therapy. Based on the combination study on ginger and garlic extract for gastric cancer, it is evident that "food is medicine and medicine is food". So, let us all use ginger and garlic paste in our recipes to prevent and mitigate cancer and related disorders. Further studies are warranted to identify if chemotherapeutic agents such as 5-FU can be consumed with ginger and garlic extracts to manage cancer and if it leads to any food-drug interaction.

# BIBLIOGRAPHY

# BIBLIOGRAPHY

Abid, N. B. S., Z. Rouis, F. Nefzi, N. Souelah and M. Aouni (2012). "Evaluation of dimethylthiazol diphenyl tetrazolium bromide and propidium iodide inclusion assays for the evaluation of cell viability by flow cytometry."

Adaki, S., R. Adaki, K. Shah and A. Karagir (2014). "Garlic: Review of literature." Indian journal of cancer **51**(4): 577.

Adams, J. M. and S. Cory (1991). "Transgenic models of tumor development." Science **254**(5035): 1161-1167.

Agrawal, D. K. and P. K. Mishra (2010). "Curcumin and its analogues: potential anticancer agents." Medicinal research reviews **30**(5): 818-860.

Ahmed, R. S., V. Seth, S. T. Pasha and B. D. Banerjee (2000). "Influence of dietary ginger (Zingiber officinales Rosc) on oxidative stress induced by malathion in rats." Food and Chemical Toxicology **38**(5): 443-450.

Ahmed, R. S., S. G. Suke, V. Seth, A. Chakraborti, A. K. Tripathi and B. D. Banerjee (2008). "Protective effects of dietary ginger (Zingiber officinales Rosc.) on lindane-induced oxidative stress in rats." Phytother Res **22**(7): 902-906.

Ajith, T. A., U. Hema and M. S. Aswathy (2007). "Zingiber officinale Roscoe prevents acetaminophen-induced acute hepatotoxicity by enhancing hepatic antioxidant status." Food and Chemical Toxicology **45**(11): 2267-2272.

Al Mofleh, I. A. (2010). "Spices, herbal xenobiotics and the stomach: friends or foes?" World J Gastroenterol **16**(22): 2710-2719.

Amagase, H., B. L. Petesch, H. Matsuura, S. Kasuga and Y. Itakura (2001). "Intake of garlic and its bioactive components." J Nutr **131**(3s): 955S-962S.

Arivazhagan, S., S. Balasenthil and S. Nagini (2000). "Garlic and neem leaf extracts enhance hepatic glutathione and glutathione dependent enzymes during N-methyl-N′-nitro-N-nitrosoguanidine (MNNG)-induced gastric carcinogenesis in rats." Phytotherapy Research **14**(4): 291-293.

Ashraf, R., K. Aamir, A. R. Shaikh and T. Ahmed (2005). "Effects of garlic on dyslipidemia in patients with type 2 diabetes mellitus." J Ayub Med Coll Abbottabad **17**(3): 60-64.

Banerjee, S. K. and S. K. Maulik (2002). "Effect of garlic on cardiovascular disorders: a review." Nutr J **1**: 4.

Barranco, S., C. Townsend, C. Casartelli, B. Macik, N. Burger, W. Boerwinkle and W. Gourley (1983). "Establishment and characterization of an in vitro model system for human adenocarcinoma of the stomach." Cancer research **43**(4): 1703-1709.

Barrera, G. (2012). "Oxidative stress and lipid peroxidation products in cancer progression and therapy." ISRN oncology **2012**.

Bayan, L., P. H. Koulivand and A. Gorji (2014). "Garlic: a review of potential therapeutic effects." Avicenna J Phytomed **4**(1): 1-14.

Bearden, M. M., D. A. Pearson, D. Rein, K. A. Chevaux, D. R. Carpenter, C. L. Keen and H. Schmitz (2000). Potential cardiovascular health benefits of procyanidins present in chocolate and cocoa, ACS Publications.

Benzie, I. F. and J. J. Strain (1996). "The ferric reducing ability of plasma (FRAP) as a measure of "antioxidant power": the FRAP assay." Anal Biochem **239**(1): 70-76.

Benzie, I. F. and J. J. Strain (1996). "The ferric reducing ability of plasma (FRAP) as a measure of "antioxidant power": the FRAP assay." Analytical biochemistry **239**(1): 70-76.

Beyer, R. E. (1994). "The role of ascorbate in antioxidant protection of biomembranes: interaction with vitamin E and coenzyme Q." Journal of bioenergetics and biomembranes **26**(4): 349-358.

Bhatia, M., K. L. McGrath, G. Di Trapani, P. Charoentong, F. Shah, M. M. King, F. M. Clarke and K. F. Tonissen (2016). "The thioredoxin system in breast cancer cell invasion and migration." Redox biology **8**: 68-78.

Bild, A. H., G. Yao, J. T. Chang, Q. Wang, A. Potti, D. Chasse, M.-B. Joshi, D. Harpole, J. M. Lancaster and A. Berchuck (2006). "Oncogenic pathway signatures in human cancers as a guide to targeted therapies." Nature **439**(7074): 353.

Bonetta, L. (2005). Prime time for real-time PCR, Nature Publishing Group.

Brahmbhatt, M., S. R. Gundala, G. Asif, S. A. Shamsi and R. Aneja (2013). "Ginger phytochemicals exhibit synergy to inhibit prostate cancer cell proliferation." Nutrition and cancer **65**(2): 263-272.

Bråkenhielm, E., R. Cao and Y. Cao (2001). "Suppression of angiogenesis, tumor growth, and wound healing by resveratrol, a natural compound in red wine and grapes." The FASEB Journal **15**(10): 1798-1800.

Brenner, H., D. Rothenbacher and V. Arndt (2009). "Epidemiology of stomach cancer." Methods Mol Biol **472**: 467-477.

Burley, S. K., H. M. Berman, C. Christie, J. M. Duarte, Z. Feng, J. Westbrook, J. Young and C. Zardecki (2018). "RCSB Protein Data Bank: Sustaining a living digital data resource that enables breakthroughs in scientific research and biomedical education." Protein Science **27**(1): 316-330.

Burstein, H. J. (2000). "Side effects of chemotherapy." Journal of Clinical Oncology **18**(3): 693-693.

Cao, A.-L., Q.-F. Tang, W.-C. Zhou, Y.-Y. Qiu, S.-J. Hu and P.-H. Yin (2015). "Ras/ERK signaling pathway is involved in curcumin-induced cell cycle arrest and apoptosis in human gastric carcinoma AGS cells." Journal of Asian natural products research **17**(1): 56-63.

Capasso, A. (2013). "Antioxidant action and therapeutic efficacy of Allium sativum L." Molecules **18**(1): 690-700.

Cekanova, M. and K. Rathore (2014). "Animal models and therapeutic molecular targets of cancer: utility and limitations." Drug design, development and therapy **8**: 1911.

Cekanova, M., M. J. Uddin, J. W. Bartges, A. Callens, A. M. Legendre, K. Rathore, L. Wright, A. Carter and L. J. Marnett (2013). "Molecular imaging of cyclooxygenase-2 in canine transitional cell carcinomas in vitro and in vivo." Cancer prevention research **6**(5): 466-476.

Cerella, C., M. Dicato, C. Jacob and M. Diederich (2011). "Chemical properties and mechanisms determining the anti-cancer action of garlic-derived organic sulfur compounds." Anti-Cancer Agents in Medicinal Chemistry (Formerly Current Medicinal Chemistry-Anti-Cancer Agents) **11**(3): 267-271.

Chabner, B. A. and T. G. Roberts Jr (2005). "Chemotherapy and the war on cancer." Nature Reviews Cancer **5**(1): 65.

Chai, E. Z. P., M. K. Shanmugam, F. Arfuso, A. Dharmarajan, C. Wang, A. P. Kumar, R. P. Samy, L. H. Lim, L. Wang and B. C. Goh (2016). "Targeting transcription factor STAT3 for cancer prevention and therapy." Pharmacology & therapeutics **162**: 86-97.

Chakraborty, D., K. Bishayee, S. Ghosh, R. Biswas, S. Kumar Mandal and A. Rahman Khuda-Bukhsh (2012). "[6]-Gingerol induces caspase 3 dependent apoptosis and autophagy in cancer cells: Drug–DNA interaction and expression of certain signal genes in HeLa cells." European Journal of Pharmacology **694**(1): 20-29.

Chan, J. Y., A. C. Yuen, R. Y. Chan and S. W. Chan (2013). "A review of the cardiovascular benefits and antioxidant properties of allicin." Phytother Res **27**(5): 637-646.

Chatterjee, P. K., N. S. Patel, E. O. Kvale, S. Cuzzocrea, P. A. Brown, K. N. Stewart, H. Mota-Filipe and C. Thiemermann (2002). "Inhibition of inducible nitric oxide synthase reduces renal ischemia/reperfusion injury." Kidney international **61**(3): 862-871.

Chen, C., D. Pung, V. Leong, V. Hebbar, G. Shen, S. Nair, W. Li and A. N. Tony Kong (2004). "Induction of detoxifying enzymes by garlic organosulfur compounds through transcription factor Nrf2: effect of chemical structure and stress signals." Free Radical Biology and Medicine **37**(10): 1578-1590.

Chen, F., H. Li, Y. Wang, M. Gao, Y. Cheng, D. Liu, M. Jia and J. Zhang (2016). "Inhibition of allicin in Eca109 and EC9706 cells via G2/M phase arrest and mitochondrial apoptosis pathway." Journal of Functional Foods **25**: 523-536.

Chen, J. (1992). "The antimutagenic and anticarcinogenic effects of tea, garlic and other natural foods in China: a review." Biomedical and environmental sciences: BES **5**(1): 1.

Chen, L. B. (1988). "Mitochondrial membrane potential in living cells." Annual review of cell biology **4**(1): 155-181.

Chen, M., A. D. Guerrero, L. Huang, Z. Shabier, M. Pan, T.-H. Tan and J. Wang (2007). "Caspase-9-induced mitochondrial disruption through cleavage of anti-apoptotic BCL-2 family members." Journal of Biological Chemistry **282**(46): 33888-33895.

Choi, J.-I., I. Joo and J. M. Lee (2014). "State-of-the-art preoperative staging of gastric cancer by MDCT and magnetic resonance imaging." World Journal of Gastroenterology: WJG **20**(16): 4546.

Choi, Y. H. (2017). "Diallyl trisulfide induces apoptosis and mitotic arrest in AGS human gastric carcinoma cells through reactive oxygen species-mediated activation of AMP-activated protein kinase." Biomedicine & Pharmacotherapy **94**: 63-71.

Chomczynski, P. and K. Mackey (1995). "Short technical reports. Modification of the TRI reagent procedure for isolation of RNA from polysaccharide-and proteoglycan-rich sources." Biotechniques **19**(6): 942-945.

Chou, T.-C. (2006). "Theoretical basis, experimental design, and computerized simulation of synergism and antagonism in drug combination studies." Pharmacological reviews **58**(3): 621-681.

Chou, T.-C. and P. Talalay (1984). "Quantitative analysis of dose-effect relationships: the combined effects of multiple drugs or enzyme inhibitors." Advances in enzyme regulation **22**: 27-55.

Citronberg, J., R. Bostick, T. Ahearn, D. K. Turgeon, M. T. Ruffin, Z. Djuric, A. Sen, D. E. Brenner and S. M. Zick (2013). "Effects of ginger supplementation on cell-cycle biomarkers in the normal-appearing colonic mucosa of patients at increased risk for colorectal cancer: results from a pilot, randomized, and controlled trial." Cancer Prevention Research.

Correa, P., M. B. Piazuelo and M. C. Camargo (2004). "The future of gastric cancer prevention." Gastric Cancer **7**(1): 9-16.

Craig, W. and L. Beck (1999). "Phytochemicals: Health Protective Effects." Can J Diet Pract Res **60**(2): 78-84.

Crowley, L. C., B. J. Marfell, A. P. Scott and N. J. Waterhouse (2016). "Quantitation of apoptosis and necrosis by annexin V binding, propidium iodide uptake, and flow cytometry." Cold Spring Harbor Protocols **2016**(11): pdb. prot087288.

Cury-Boaventura, M. F., C. Pompéia and R. Curi (2004). "Comparative toxicity of oleic acid and linoleic acid on Jurkat cells." Clinical nutrition **23**(4): 721-732.

da Silva, J. A., A. B. Becceneri, H. S. Mutti, A. C. B. M. Martin, J. B. Fernandes, P. C. Vieira and M. R. Cominetti (2012). "Purification and differential biological effects of ginger-derived substances on normal and tumor cell lines." Journal of Chromatography B **903**: 157-162.

Danwilai, K., J. Konmun, B.-o. Sripanidkulchai and S. Subongkot (2017). "Antioxidant activity of ginger extract as a daily supplement in cancer patients receiving adjuvant chemotherapy: a pilot study." Cancer Management and Research **9**: 11-18.

Das, T. P., S. Suman and C. Damodaran (2014). "Induction of reactive oxygen species generation inhibits epithelial–mesenchymal transition and promotes growth arrest in prostate cancer cells." Molecular carcinogenesis **53**(7): 537-547.

Dethier, B., M. Laloux, E. Hanon, K. Nott, S. Heuskin and J.-P. Wathelet (2012). "Analysis of the diastereoisomers of alliin by HPLC." Talanta **101**: 447-452.

Dicken, B. J., D. L. Bigam, C. Cass, J. R. Mackey, A. A. Joy and S. M. Hamilton (2005). "Gastric adenocarcinoma: review and considerations for future directions." Annals of surgery **241**(1): 27.

Dickins, R. A., K. McJunkin, E. Hernando, P. K. Premsrirut, V. Krizhanovsky, D. J. Burgess, S. Y. Kim, C. Cordon-Cardo, L. Zender and G. J. Hannon (2007). "Tissue-specific and reversible RNA interference in transgenic mice." Nature genetics **39**(7): 914.

Dikshit, R. P., G. Mathur, S. Mhatre and B. Yeole (2011). "Epidemiological review of gastric cancer in India." Indian journal of medical and paediatric oncology: official journal of Indian Society of Medical & Paediatric Oncology **32**(1): 3.

Dixon, K. and E. Kopras (2004). Genetic alterations and DNA repair in human carcinogenesis. Seminars in cancer biology, Elsevier.

Drews, J. (2000). "Drug discovery: a historical perspective." Science **287**(5460): 1960-1964.

Ekambaram, G., P. Rajendran, V. Magesh and D. Sakthisekaran (2008). "Naringenin reduces tumor size and weight lost in N-methyl-N′-nitro-N-nitrosoguanidine–induced gastric carcinogenesis in rats." Nutrition Research **28**(2): 106-112.

Elmore, S. (2007). "Apoptosis: a review of programmed cell death." Toxicologic pathology **35**(4): 495-516.

ElRokh, E.-S. M., N. A. Yassin, S. M. El-Shenawy and B. M. Ibrahim (2010). "Antihypercholesterolaemic effect of ginger rhizome (Zingiber officinale) in rats." Inflammopharmacology **18**(6): 309-315.

Fan, J., X. Yang and Z. Bi (2015). "6-Gingerol inhibits osteosarcoma cell proliferation through apoptosis and AMPK activation." Tumor Biology **36**(2): 1135-1141.

Ferrand, A. and T. C. Wang (2006). "Gastrin and cancer: a review." Cancer letters **238**(1): 15-29.

Ferrandez, A., S. Prescott and R. W. Burt (2003). "COX-2 and colorectal cancer." Curr Pharm Des **9**(27): 2229-2251.

Forones, N. M., A. P. S. Carvalho, O. Giannotti-Filho, L. G. Lourenço and C. T. F. Oshima (2005). "Cell proliferation and apoptosis in gastric cancer and intestinal metaplasia." Arquivos de gastroenterologia **42**(1): 30-34.

Fox, J. G. and T. C. Wang (2007). "Inflammation, atrophy, and gastric cancer." The Journal of clinical investigation **117**(1): 60-69.

Frese, K. K. and D. A. Tuveson (2007). "Maximizing mouse cancer models." Nature Reviews Cancer **7**(9): 654.

Fujimoto-Ouchi, K., F. Sekiguchi, H. Yasuno, Y. Moriya, K. Mori and Y. Tanaka (2007). "Antitumor activity of trastuzumab in combination with chemotherapy in human gastric cancer xenograft models." Cancer chemotherapy and pharmacology **59**(6): 795-805.

Fulda, S., L. Galluzzi and G. Kroemer (2010). "Targeting mitochondria for cancer therapy." Nature reviews Drug discovery 9(6): 447.

Fulda, S. and D. Kögel (2015). "Cell death by autophagy: emerging molecular mechanisms and implications for cancer therapy." Oncogene 34(40): 5105.

Gallorini, M., A. Cataldi and V. di Giacomo (2012). "Cyclin-dependent kinase modulators and cancer therapy." BioDrugs 26(6): 377-391.

Gauthé, M., M. Richard-Molard, W. Cacheux, P. Michel, J.-L. Jouve, E. Mitry, J.-L. Alberini and A. Lièvre (2015). "Role of fluorine 18 fluorodeoxyglucose positron emission tomography/computed tomography in gastrointestinal cancers." Digestive and Liver Disease 47(6): 443-454.

Gill, S. S. and N. Tuteja (2010). "Reactive oxygen species and antioxidant machinery in abiotic stress tolerance in crop plants." Plant physiology and biochemistry 48(12): 909-930.

Glatthaar, B. E., D. H. Hornig and U. Moser (1986). "The role of ascorbic acid in carcinogenesis." Adv Exp Med Biol 206: 357-377.

González, C. A., P. Jakszyn, G. Pera, A. Agudo, S. Bingham, D. Palli, P. Ferrari, H. Boeing, G. Del Giudice and M. Plebani (2006). "Meat intake and risk of stomach and esophageal adenocarcinoma within the European Prospective Investigation Into Cancer and Nutrition (EPIC)." Journal of the National Cancer Institute 98(5): 345-354.

Gossen, M. and H. Bujard (1992). "Tight control of gene expression in mammalian cells by tetracycline-responsive promoters." Proceedings of the National Academy of Sciences 89(12): 5547-5551.

Grogan, T. M., C. Fenoglio-Prieser, R. Zeheb, W. Bellamy, Y. Frutiger, E. Vela, G. Stemmerman, J. Macdonald, L. Richter, A. Gallegos and G. Powis (2000). "Thioredoxin, a putative oncogene product,is overexpressed in gastric carcinoma and associated with increased proliferation and increased cell survival." Human Pathology 31(4): 475-481.

Gross, A., J. M. McDonnell and S. J. Korsmeyer (1999). "BCL-2 family members and the mitochondria in apoptosis." Genes & development 13(15): 1899-1911.

Grzanna, R., L. Lindmark and C. G. Frondoza (2005). "Ginger—an herbal medicinal product with broad anti-inflammatory actions." Journal of medicinal food 8(2): 125-132.

Gudarzi, H., M. Salimi, S. Irian, A. Amanzadeh, H. Mostafapour Kandelous, K. Azadmanesh and M. Salimi (2015). "Ethanolic extract of Ferula gummosa is cytotoxic against cancer cells by inducing apoptosis and cell cycle arrest." Natural Product Research 29(6): 546-550.

Guilford, W. G. (1990). "Upper gastrointestinal endoscopy." Veterinary Clinics of North America: Small Animal Practice 20(5): 1209-1227.

Guo, X.-y., G.-f. Sun and Y.-c. Sun (2003). "Oxidative stress from fluoride-induced hepatotoxicity in rats." Fluoride **36**(1): 25-29.

Gupta, M. (2010). "Pharmacological properties and traditional therapeutic uses of important Indian spices: A review." International Journal of Food Properties **13**(5): 1092-1116.

Habig, W. H., M. J. Pabst and W. B. Jakoby (1974). "Glutathione S-transferases the first enzymatic step in mercapturic acid formation." Journal of biological Chemistry **249**(22): 7130-7139.

Hall, A. (1999). "The role of glutathione in the regulation of apoptosis." European journal of clinical investigation **29**: 238-245.

Halldórsdóttir, A. M., M. Sigurdardóttir, J. G. Jónasson, M. Oddsdóttir, J. Magnússon, J. R. Lee and J. R. Goldenring (2003). "Spasmolytic polypeptide-expressing metaplasia (SPEM) associated with gastric cancer in Iceland." Digestive diseases and sciences **48**(3): 431-441.

Hallemeier, C. L. and M. G. Haddock (2017). Gastric Cancer: Radiation Therapy Planning. Radiation Therapy for Gastrointestinal Cancers, Springer: 59-71.

Halliwell, B. (1995). "Antioxidant characterization: methodology and mechanism." Biochemical pharmacology **49**(10): 1341-1348.

Halliwell, B. (1995). "How to characterize an antioxidant: an update." Biochem Soc Symp **61**: 73-101.

Halvorsen, B. L., K. Holte, M. C. Myhrstad, I. Barikmo, E. Hvattum, S. F. Remberg, A.-B. Wold, K. Haffner, H. Baugerød and L. F. Andersen (2002). "A systematic screening of total antioxidants in dietary plants." The Journal of nutrition **132**(3): 461-471.

Hamzeloo-Moghadam, M., M. Aghaei, F. Fallahian, S. M. Jafari, M. Dolati, M. H. Abdolmohammadi, S. Hajiahmadi and S. Esmaeili (2015). "Britannin, a sesquiterpene lactone, inhibits proliferation and induces apoptosis through the mitochondrial signaling pathway in human breast cancer cells." Tumor Biology **36**(2): 1191-1198.

Hansen, M. B., S. E. Nielsen and K. Berg (1989). "Re-examination and further development of a precise and rapid dye method for measuring cell growth/cell kill." Journal of immunological methods **119**(2): 203-210.

Harmon, R. C. and D. A. Peura (2010). "Evaluation and management of dyspepsia." Therapeutic advances in gastroenterology **3**(2): 87-98.

Hayes, J. D., L. A. Kerr and A. D. Cronshaw (1989). "Evidence that glutathione S-transferases B1B1 and B2B2 are the products of separate genes and that their expression in human liver is subject to inter-individual variation. Molecular relationships between the B1 and B2 subunits and other Alpha class glutathione S-transferases." Biochemical Journal **264**(2): 437.

Hecht, S. S. (1999). "Chemoprevention of cancer by isothiocyanates, modifiers of carcinogen metabolism." The Journal of nutrition **129**(3): 768S-774S.

Henle, G. and F. Deinhardt (1957). "The establishment of strains of human cells in tissue culture." The Journal of Immunology **79**(1): 54-59.

Hindmarsh, J. T. and P. F. Corso (1998). "The death of Napoleon Bonaparte: a critical review of the cause." Journal of the history of medicine and allied sciences **53**(3): 201-218.

Hinz, B. and K. Brune (2002). "Cyclooxygenase-2—10 years later." Journal of Pharmacology and Experimental Therapeutics **300**(2): 367-375.

Hirsch, K., M. Danilenko, J. Giat, T. Miron, A. Rabinkov, M. Wilchek, D. Mirelman, J. Levy and Y. Sharoni (2000). "Effect of Purified Allicin, the Major Ingredient of Freshly Crushed Garlic, on Cancer Cell Proliferation." Nutrition and Cancer **38**(2): 245-254.

Hiserodt, R., S. Franzblau and R. Rosen (1998). "Isolation of 6-, 8-, and 10- Gingerol from Ginger Rhizome by HPLC and Preliminary Evaluation of Inhibition of Mycobacterium avium and Mycobacterium tuberculosis." Journal of agricultural and food chemistry **46**(7): 2504-2508.

Houshmand, B., F. Mahjour and O. Dianat (2013). "Antibacterial effect of different concentrations of garlic (Allium sativum) extract on dental plaque bacteria." Indian J Dent Res **24**(1): 71-75.

Hsing, A. W., A. P. Chokkalingam, Y.-T. Gao, M. P. Madigan, J. Deng, G. Gridley and J. F. Fraumeni Jr (2002). "Allium vegetables and risk of prostate cancer: a population-based study." Journal of the National Cancer Institute **94**(21): 1648-1651.

Hu, B., N. El Hajj, S. Sittler, N. Lammert, R. Barnes and A. Meloni-Ehrig (2012). "Gastric cancer: Classification, histology and application of molecular pathology." J Gastrointest Oncol **3**(3): 251-261.

Huynh, A. S., D. F. Abrahams, M. S. Torres, M. K. Baldwin, R. J. Gillies and D. L. Morse (2011). "Development of an orthotopic human pancreatic cancer xenograft model using ultrasound guided injection of cells." PloS one **6**(5): e20330.

Jacks, T., A. Fazeli, E. M. Schmitt, R. T. Bronson, M. A. Goodell and R. A. Weinberg (1992). "Effects of an Rb mutation in the mouse." Nature **359**(6393): 295.

Jakszyn, P. and C. A. González (2006). "Nitrosamine and related food intake and gastric and oesophageal cancer risk: a systematic review of the epidemiological evidence." World journal of gastroenterology: WJG **12**(27): 4296.

Kakkar, P., B. Das and P. Viswanathan (1984). "A modified spectrophotometric assay of superoxide dismutase."

Kam, P. and N. Ferch (2000). "Apoptosis: mechanisms and clinical implications." Anaesthesia **55**(11): 1081-1093.

Kapetanovic, I. (2008). "Computer-aided drug discovery and development (CADDD): in silico-chemico-biological approach." Chemico-biological interactions **171**(2): 165-176.

Karimi, N. and V. D. Roshan (2013). "Change in adiponectin and oxidative stress after modifiable lifestyle interventions in breast cancer cases." Asian Pac J Cancer Prev **14**(5): 2845-2850.

Karlenius, T. C. and K. F. Tonissen (2010). "Thioredoxin and cancer: a role for thioredoxin in all states of tumor oxygenation." Cancers 2(2): 209-232.

Karuppiah, P. and S. Rajaram (2012). "Antibacterial effect of Allium sativum cloves and Zingiber officinale rhizomes against multiple-drug resistant clinical pathogens." Asian Pac J Trop Biomed 2(8): 597-601.

Kaschula, C. H., R. Hunter and M. I. Parker (2010). "Garlic-derived anticancer agents: structure and biological activity of ajoene." Biofactors 36(1): 78-85.

Kastan, M. B. and J. Bartek (2004). "Cell-cycle checkpoints and cancer." Nature 432(7015): 316.

Kelley, J. R. and J. M. Duggan (2003). "Gastric cancer epidemiology and risk factors." Journal of clinical epidemiology 56(1): 1-9.

Kemp, C. J. (2015). "Animal models of chemical carcinogenesis: driving breakthroughs in cancer research for 100 years." Cold Spring Harbor Protocols 2015(10): pdb. top069906.

Kim, D.-K., S. Y. Oh, H.-C. Kwon, S. Lee, K. A. Kwon, B. G. Kim, S.-G. Kim, S.-H. Kim, J. S. Jang and M. C. Kim (2009). "Clinical significances of preoperative serum interleukin-6 and C-reactive protein level in operable gastric cancer." BMC cancer 9(1): 155.

Kim, H.-H., W. J. Hyung, G. S. Cho, M. C. Kim, S.-U. Han, W. Kim, S.-W. Ryu, H.-J. Lee and K. Y. Song (2010). "Morbidity and mortality of laparoscopic gastrectomy versus open gastrectomy for gastric cancer: an interim report—a phase III multicenter, prospective, randomized Trial (KLASS Trial)." Annals of surgery 251(3): 417-420.

Kim, K.-H., S.-J. Cho, B.-O. Kim and S. Pyo (2016). "Differential pro-apoptotic effect of allicin in oestrogen receptor-positive or -negative human breast cancer cells." Journal of Functional Foods 25: 341-353.

Klaunig, J. E. and L. M. Kamendulis (2004). "The role of oxidative stress in carcinogenesis." Annu. Rev. Pharmacol. Toxicol. 44: 239-267.

Koch, H. P. and L. D. Lawson (1996). Garlic: the science and therapeutic application of Allium sativum L. and related species, baltimore, Maryland: Williams & Wilkins xv, 329p. ISBN.

Koh, T. and T. Wang (2002). "Tumors of the stomach." Sleisenger & Fordtran's Gastrointestinal and Liver Disease. 7th ed. Philadelphia: Saunders: 829-844.

Kolev, Y., H. Uetake, Y. Takagi and K. Sugihara (2008). "Lactate dehydrogenase-5 (LDH-5) expression in human gastric cancer: association with hypoxia-inducible factor (HIF-1α) pathway, angiogenic factors production and poor prognosis." Annals of surgical oncology 15(8): 2336-2344.

Koleva, I. I., T. A. Van Beek, J. P. Linssen, A. d. Groot and L. N. Evstatieva (2002). "Screening of plant extracts for antioxidant activity: a comparative study on three testing methods." Phytochemical analysis 13(1): 8-17.

Kota, N., P. Krishna and K. Polasa (2008). "Alterations in antioxidant status of rats following intake of ginger through diet." Food Chemistry 106(3): 991-996.

Kou, X., X. Li, M. R. T. Rahman, M. Yan, H. Huang, H. Wang and Y. Su (2017). "Efficient dehydration of 6-gingerol to 6-shogaol catalyzed by an acidic ionic liquid under ultrasound irradiation." Food chemistry **215**: 193-199.

Kracht, M. (2007). "Targeting strategies to modulate the NF-κB and JNK signal transduction network." Anti-Inflammatory & Anti-Allergy Agents in Medicinal Chemistry (Formerly Current Medicinal Chemistry-Anti-Inflammatory and Anti-Allergy Agents) **6**(1): 71-84.

Kwee, R. M. and T. C. Kwee (2015). "Modern imaging techniques for preoperative detection of distant metastases in gastric cancer." World Journal of Gastroenterology: WJG **21**(37): 10502.

Kweon, S., K.-A. Park and H. Choi (2003). "Chemopreventive effect of garlic powder diet in diethylnitrosamine-induced rat hepatocarcinogenesis." Life Sciences **73**(19): 2515-2526.

Labianca, R., S. Marsoni, G. Pancera, V. Torri, A. Zaniboni, C. Erlichman, J. Pater, L. Shepherd, B. Zee and J. Seitz (1995). "Efficacy of adjuvant fluorouracil and folinic acid in colon cancer." The Lancet **345**(8955): 939-944.

Lampe, J. W. (1999). "Health effects of vegetables and fruit: assessing mechanisms of action in human experimental studies." The American journal of clinical nutrition **70**(3): 475s-490s.

Lantz, R. C., G. J. Chen, M. Sarihan, A. M. Solyom, S. D. Jolad and B. N. Timmermann (2007). "The effect of extracts from ginger rhizome on inflammatory mediator production." Phytomedicine **14**(2-3): 123-128.

Lawrence, T. (2009). "The nuclear factor NF-kappaB pathway in inflammation." Cold Spring Harb Perspect Biol **1**(6): a001651.

Lee, C.-H., H.-C. Huang and H.-F. Juan (2011). "Reviewing ligand-based rational drug design: The search for an ATP synthase inhibitor." International journal of molecular sciences **12**(8): 5304-5318.

Lee, C. G., H.-W. Lee, B.-O. Kim, D.-K. Rhee and S. Pyo (2015). "Allicin inhibits invasion and migration of breast cancer cells through the suppression of VCAM-1: Regulation of association between p65 and ER-α." Journal of Functional Foods **15**: 172-185.

Lee, D.-H., D.-W. Kim, C.-H. Jung, Y. J. Lee and D. Park (2014). "Gingerol sensitizes TRAIL-induced apoptotic cell death of glioblastoma cells." Toxicology and applied pharmacology **279**(3): 253-265.

Lee, H. S., E. Y. Seo, N. E. Kang and W. K. Kim (2008). "[6]-Gingerol inhibits metastasis of MDA-MB-231 human breast cancer cells." The Journal of nutritional biochemistry **19**(5): 313-319.

Lee, J., S. Gupta, J.-S. Huang, L. P. Jayathilaka and B.-S. Lee (2013). "HPLC–MTT assay: Anticancer activity of aqueous garlic extract is from allicin." Analytical biochemistry **436**(2): 187-189.

Leung, W. K., K.-c. Wu, C. Y. Wong, A. S. Cheng, A. K. Ching, A. W. Chan, W. W.

Chong, M. Y. Go, J. Yu and K.-F. To (2008). "Transgenic cyclooxygenase-2 expression and high salt enhanced susceptibility to chemical-induced gastric cancer development in mice." Carcinogenesis **29**(8): 1648-1654.

Leung, W. K., M.-s. Wu, Y. Kakugawa, J. J. Kim, K.-g. Yeoh, K. L. Goh, K.-c. Wu, D.-c. Wu, J. Sollano and U. Kachintorn (2008). "Screening for gastric cancer in Asia: current evidence and practice." The lancet oncology **9**(3): 279-287.

Lewis, G. D., S. B. Chiang, E. B. Butler and B. S. Teh (2017). "The utility of positron emission tomography/computed tomography in target delineation for stereotactic body radiotherapy for liver metastasis from primary gastric cancer: an illustrative case report and literature review." Journal of Gastrointestinal Oncology.

Li, C., H. Jing, G. Ma and P. Liang (2018). "Allicin induces apoptosis through activation of both intrinsic and extrinsic pathways in glioma cells." Molecular medicine reports.

Li, Z. (2011). "In Vitro Micro-Tissue and-Organ Models for Toxicity Testing."

Liang, C.-C., A. Y. Park and J.-L. Guan (2007). "In vitro scratch assay: a convenient and inexpensive method for analysis of cell migration in vitro." Nature protocols **2**(2): 329.

Lifshitz, S., S. A. Lamprecht, D. Benharroch, I. Prinsloo, S. Polak-Charcon and B. Schwartz (2001). "Apoptosis (programmed cell death) in colonic cells: from normal to transformed stage." Cancer letters **163**(2): 229-238.

Lim, J. W., H. Kim and K. H. Kim (2001). "Nuclear factor-kappaB regulates cyclooxygenase-2 expression and cell proliferation in human gastric cancer cells." Lab Invest **81**(3): 349-360.

Lin, W. W. and M. Karin (2007). "A cytokine-mediated link between innate immunity, inflammation, and cancer." J Clin Invest **117**(5): 1175-1183.

Ling, L., K. Tan, H. Lin and G. Chiu (2011). "The role of reactive oxygen species and autophagy in safingol-induced cell death." Cell death & disease **2**(3): e129.

Liou, G.-Y. and P. Storz (2010). "Reactive oxygen species in cancer." Free radical research **44**(5): 479-496.

Liu, K., P.-c. Liu, R. Liu and X. Wu (2015). "Dual AO/EB staining to detect apoptosis in osteosarcoma cells compared with flow cytometry." Medical science monitor basic research **21**: 15.

Liu, T., A. Stern, L. J. Roberts and J. D. Morrow (1999). "The isoprostanes: novel prostaglandin-like products of the free radical-catalyzed peroxidation of arachidonic acid." J Biomed Sci **6**(4): 226-235.

Liu, Y., T. Yin, Y. Feng, M. M. Cona, G. Huang, J. Liu, S. Song, Y. Jiang, Q. Xia and J. V. Swinnen (2015). "Mammalian models of chemically induced primary malignancies exploitable for imaging-based preclinical theragnostic research." Quantitative imaging in medicine and surgery **5**(5): 708.

Lobo, V., A. Patil, A. Phatak and N. Chandra (2010). "Free radicals, antioxidants and functional foods:

Impact on human health." Pharmacognosy Reviews **4**(8): 118-126.

Longley, D. B., D. P. Harkin and P. G. Johnston (2003). "5-fluorouracil: mechanisms of action and clinical strategies." Nature Reviews Cancer **3**(5): 330.

Ma, D.-L., D. S.-H. Chan and C.-H. Leung (2011). "Molecular docking for virtual screening of natural product databases." Chemical Science **2**(9): 1656-1665.

Makarov, S. S. (2000). "NF-κB as a therapeutic target in chronic inflammation: recent advances." Molecular medicine today **6**(11): 441-448.

Manju, V. and N. Nalini (2005). "Chemopreventive efficacy of ginger, a naturally occurring anticarcinogen during the initiation, post-initiation stages of 1,2 dimethylhydrazine-induced colon cancer." Clin Chim Acta **358**(1-2): 60-67.

Mantovani, A., P. Allavena, A. Sica and F. Balkwill (2008). "Cancer-related inflammation." Nature **454**(7203): 436.

Manuel del Casar, J., F. J. Vizoso, O. Abdel-Laa, L. Sanz, A. Martín, M. Daniela Corte, M. Bongera, J. L. García Muñiz and A. Fueyo (2004). "Prognostic value of cytosolyc cathepsin D content in resectable gastric cancer." Journal of surgical oncology **86**(1): 16-21.

Marcus, C. and R. M. Subramaniam (2017). "PET/Computed Tomography and Precision Medicine." PET clinics **12**(4): 437-447.

Marnett, L. J. (1999). "Lipid peroxidation—DNA damage by malondialdehyde." Mutation Research/Fundamental and Molecular Mechanisms of Mutagenesis **424**(1): 83-95.

Mathew, A., P. Gangadharan, C. Varghese and M. K. Nair (2000). "Diet and stomach cancer: a case-control study in South India." Eur J Cancer Prev **9**(2): 89-97.

Mattar, R., C. R. A. d. Andrade, G. M. DiFavero, J. J. Gama-Rodrigues and A. A. Laudanna (2002). "Preoperative serum levels of CA 72-4, CEA, CA 19-9, and alpha-fetoprotein in patients with gastric cancer." Revista do Hospital das Clínicas **57**(3): 89-92.

McCord, J. M. and I. Fridovich (1969). "The utility of superoxide dismutase in studying free radical reactions I. radicals generated by the interaction of sulfite, dimethyl sulfoxide, and oxygen." Journal of Biological Chemistry **244**(22): 6056-6063.

Miki, K., T. Oda, J. Miyazaki, S. Iino, H. Niwa, H. Oka and S. Suzuki (1980). "Alkaline phosphatase isoenzymes in intestinal metaplasia and carcinoma of rat stomach induced by N-methyl-N'-nitro-N-nitrosoguanidine." Oncodevelopmental biology and medicine: the journal of the International Society for Oncodevelopmental Biology and Medicine **1**(4-5): 313-323.

Misra, V., R. Pandey, S. P. Misra and M. Dwivedi (2014). "Helicobacter pylori and gastric cancer: Indian enigma." World Journal of Gastroenterology: WJG **20**(6): 1503.

Morton, C. L. and P. J. Houghton (2007). "Establishment of human tumor xenografts in immunodeficient mice." Nature protocols **2**(2): 247.

Mosmann, T. (1983). "Rapid colorimetric assay for cellular growth and survival: application to proliferation and cytotoxicity assays." Journal of immunological methods **65**(1-2): 55-63.

Munday, R. and C. M. Munday (2001). "Relative activities of organosulfur compounds derived from onions and garlic in increasing tissue activities of quinone reductase and glutathione transferase in rat tissues." Nutrition and cancer **40**(2): 205-210.

Murphy, M. P., A. Holmgren, N.-G. Larsson, B. Halliwell, C. J. Chang, B. Kalyanaraman, S. G. Rhee, P. J. Thornalley, L. Partridge and D. Gems (2011). "Unraveling the biological roles of reactive oxygen species." Cell metabolism **13**(4): 361-366.

Nakajima, T. (2005). Historical review of research and treatment of gastric cancer in Japan: clinical aspect. The diversity of gastric carcinoma, Springer: 29-47.

Nammi, S., Y.-T. Sun and D. Chang (2014). "Effects of Ginger on Metabolic Syndrome." Clinical Aspects of Functional Foods and Nutraceuticals: 381.

Nasr, A. Y. (2014). "Protective effect of aged garlic extract against the oxidative stress induced by cisplatin on blood cells parameters and hepatic antioxidant enzymes in rats." Toxicology Reports **1**: 682-691.

Navarro, J., E. Obrador, J. Carretero, I. Petschen, J. Avino, P. Perez and J. M. Estrela (1999). "Changes in glutathione status and the antioxidant system in blood and in cancer cells associate with tumour growth in vivo." Free Radical Biology and Medicine **26**(3): 410-418.

Navarro, J., E. Obrador, J. A. Pellicer, M. Asensi, J. Viña and J. M. Estrela (1997). "Blood glutathione as an index of radiation-induced oxidative stress in mice and humans." Free Radical Biology and Medicine **22**(7): 1203-1209.

Nicastro, H. L., S. A. Ross and J. A. Milner (2015). "Garlic and onions: their cancer prevention properties." Cancer Prev Res (Phila) **8**(3): 181-189.

Niccolai, E., A. Taddei, D. Prisco and A. Amedei (2015). "Gastric cancer and the epoch of immunotherapy approaches." World Journal of Gastroenterology: WJG **21**(19): 5778.

Nicolini, A., P. Ferrari, M. C. Masoni, M. Fini, S. Pagani, O. Giampietro and A. Carpi (2013). "Malnutrition, anorexia and cachexia in cancer patients: a mini-review on pathogenesis and treatment." Biomedicine & Pharmacotherapy **67**(8): 807-817.

Nielsen, F., B. B. Mikkelsen, J. B. Nielsen, H. R. Andersen and P. Grandjean (1997). "Plasma malondialdehyde as biomarker for oxidative stress: reference interval and effects of life-style factors." Clinical chemistry **43**(7): 1209-1214.

Nigam, N., K. Bhui, S. Prasad, J. George and Y. Shukla (2009). "[6]-Gingerol induces reactive oxygen species regulated mitochondrial cell death pathway in human epidermoid carcinoma A431 cells." Chemico-Biological Interactions **181**(1): 77-84.

Nozoe, T., E. Mori, I. Takahashi and T. Ezaki (2008). "Preoperative elevation of serum C-reactive protein as an independent prognostic indicator of colorectal carcinoma." Surgery today 38(7): 597-602.

Oda, I., T. Gotoda, H. Hamanaka, T. Eguchi, Y. Saito, T. Matsuda, P. Bhandari, F. Emura, D. Saito and H. Ono (2005). "Endoscopic submucosal dissection for early gastric cancer: technical feasibility, operation time and complications from a large consecutive series." Digestive endoscopy 17(1): 54-58.

Ohkawa, H., N. Ohishi and K. Yagi (1979). "Assay for lipid peroxides in animal tissues by thiobarbituric acid reaction." Analytical biochemistry 95(2): 351-358.

Omar, S. and N. Al-Wabel (2010). "Organosulfur compounds and possible mechanism of garlic in cancer." Saudi Pharmaceutical Journal 18(1): 51-58.

Omaye, S. T., J. D. Turnbull and H. E. Sauberlich (1979). [1] Selected methods for the determination of ascorbic acid in animal cells, tissues, and fluids. Methods in enzymology, Elsevier. 62: 3-11.

Orditura, M., G. Galizia, V. Sforza, V. Gambardella, A. Fabozzi, M. M. Laterza, F. Andreozzi, J. Ventriglia, B. Savastano and A. Mabilia (2014). "Treatment of gastric cancer." World journal of gastroenterology: WJG 20(7): 1635.

Padiya, R. and S. K. Banerjee (2013). "Garlic as an anti-diabetic agent: recent progress and patent reviews." Recent Pat Food Nutr Agric 5(2): 105-127.

Pan, M. H., M. C. Hsieh, J. M. Kuo, C. S. Lai, H. Wu, S. Sang and C. T. Ho (2008). "6-Shogaol induces apoptosis in human colorectal carcinoma cells via ROS production, caspase activation, and GADD 153 expression." Molecular nutrition & food research 52(5): 527-537.

Pari, L. and K. Amudha (2011). "Antioxidant effect of naringin on nickel-induced toxicity in rats: an in vivo and in vitro study." International Journal of Pharmaceutical Sciences and Research 2(1): 137.

Park, Y. J., J. Wen, S. Bang, S. W. Park and S. Y. Song (2006). "[6]-Gingerol induces cell cycle arrest and cell death of mutant p53-expressing pancreatic cancer cells." Yonsei medical journal 47(5): 688-697.

Pashaei-Asl, R., F. Pashaei-Asl, P. Mostafa Gharabaghi, K. Khodadadi, M. Ebrahimi, E. Ebrahimie and M. Pashaiasl (2017). "The Inhibitory Effect of Ginger Extract on Ovarian Cancer Cell Line; Application of Systems Biology." Advanced Pharmaceutical Bulletin 7(2): 241-249.

Pavithran, K., D. C. Doval and K. K. Pandey (2002). "Gastric cancer in India." Gastric Cancer 5(4): 0240-0243.

Pelucchi, C., N. Lunet, S. Boccia, Z.-F. Zhang, D. Praud, P. Boffetta, F. Levi, K. Matsuo, H. Ito and J. Hu (2015). "The stomach cancer pooling (StoP) project: study design and presentation." European Journal of Cancer Prevention 24(1): 16-23.

Peng, F., Q. Tao, X. Wu, H. Dou, S. Spencer, C. Mang, L. Xu, L. Sun, Y. Zhao and H. Li (2012). "Cytotoxic, cytoprotective and antioxidant effects of isolated phenolic compounds from fresh ginger." Fitoterapia 83(3): 568-585.

Peng, K.-T., W.-H. Hsu, H.-N. Shih, C.-W. Hsieh, T.-W. Huang, R.-W. Hsu and P.-J. Chang (2011). "The role of reactive oxygen species scavenging enzymes in the development of septic loosening after total hip replacement." J Bone Joint Surg Br **93**(9): 1201-1209.

Pérez-Severiano, F., M. Rodríguez-Pérez, J. Pedraza-Chaverrí, P. D. Maldonado, O. N. Medina-Campos, A. Ortíz-Plata, A. Sánchez-García, J. Villeda-Hernández, S. Galván-Arzate and P. Aguilera (2004). "S-Allylcysteine, a garlic-derived antioxidant, ameliorates quinolinic acid-induced neurotoxicity and oxidative damage in rats." Neurochemistry international **45**(8): 1175-1183.

Pervin, S., R. Singh and G. Chaudhuri (2001). "Nitric oxide-induced cytostasis and cell cycle arrest of a human breast cancer cell line (MDA-MB-231): potential role of cyclin D1." Proceedings of the National Academy of Sciences **98**(6): 3583-3588.

Pestova, K., A. J. Koch, C. P. Quesenberry, J. Shan, Y. Zhang, A. D. Leimpeter, B. Blondin, S. Sitailo, L. Buckingham and J. Du (2018). "Identification of fluorescence in situ hybridization assay markers for prediction of disease progression in prostate cancer patients on active surveillance." BMC cancer **18**(1): 2.

Petrova, Y. I., L. Schecterson and B. M. Gumbiner (2016). "Roles for E-cadherin cell surface regulation in cancer." Molecular biology of the cell **27**(21): 3233-3244.

Pine, S. R., L. E. Mechanic, L. Enewold, A. K. Chaturvedi, H. A. Katki, Y.-L. Zheng, E. D. Bowman, E. A. Engels, N. E. Caporaso and C. C. Harris (2011). "Increased Levels of Circulating Interleukin 6, Interleukin 8, C-Reactive Protein, and Risk of Lung Cancer." JNCI: Journal of the National Cancer Institute **103**(14): 1112-1122.

Poh, A. R., R. J. O'donoghue, M. Ernst and T. L. Putoczki (2016). "Mouse models for gastric cancer: Matching models to biological questions." Journal of gastroenterology and hepatology **31**(7): 1257-1272.

Polterauer, S., C. Grimm, C. Tempfer, G. Sliutz, P. Speiser, A. Reinthaller and L. A. Hefler (2007). "C-reactive protein is a prognostic parameter in patients with cervical cancer." Gynecologic oncology **107**(1): 114-117.

Poprac, P., K. Jomova, M. Simunkova, V. Kollar, C. J. Rhodes and M. Valko (2017). "Targeting free radicals in oxidative stress-related human diseases." Trends in pharmacological sciences **38**(7): 592-607.

Prati, P., C. M. Henrique, A. S. d. Souza, V. S. N. d. Silva and M. T. B. Pacheco (2014). "Evaluation of allicin stability in processed garlic of different cultivars." Food Science and Technology **34**(3): 623-628.

Qin, J., M. Liu, Q. Ding, X. Ji, Y. Hao, X. Wu and J. Xiong (2014). "The direct effect of estrogen on cell viability and apoptosis in human gastric cancer cells." Molecular and cellular biochemistry **395**(1-2): 99-107.

Račková, L., M. Cupáková, A. Ťažký, J. Mičová, E. Kolek and D. Košťálová (2013). "Redox properties of ginger extracts: Perspectives of use of Zingiber officinale Rosc. as antidiabetic agent." Interdisciplinary Toxicology 6(1): 26-33.

Radhakrishnan, E., S. V. Bava, S. S. Narayanan, L. R. Nath, A. K. T. Thulasidasan, E. V. Soniya and R. J. Anto (2014). "[6]-Gingerol induces caspase-dependent apoptosis and prevents PMA-induced proliferation in colon cancer cells by inhibiting MAPK/AP-1 signaling." PLoS One 9(8): e104401.

Rajesh, E., L. S. Sankari, L. Malathi and J. R. Krupaa (2015). "Naturally occurring products in cancer therapy." Journal of pharmacy & bioallied sciences 7(Suppl 1): S181.

Rani, H. S., G. Madhavi, B. Srikanth, P. Jharna, U. Rao and A. Jyothy (2006). "Serum ADA and C-reactive protein in rheumatoid arthritis." International Journal of Human Genetics 6(3): 195-198.

Rao, C. V. (2007). Regulation of COX and LOX by curcumin. The Molecular Targets and Therapeutic Uses of Curcumin in Health and Disease, Springer: 213-226.

Rastogi, N., S. Duggal, S. K. Singh, K. Porwal, V. K. Srivastava, R. Maurya, M. L. Bhatt and D. P. Mishra (2015). "Proteasome inhibition mediates p53 reactivation and anti-cancer activity of 6-gingerol in cervical cancer cells." Oncotarget 6(41): 43310.

Rastogi, N., R. K. Gara, R. Trivedi, A. Singh, P. Dixit, R. Maurya, S. Duggal, M. L. B. Bhatt, S. Singh and D. P. Mishra (2014). "(6)-Gingerolinduced myeloid leukemia cell death is initiated by reactive oxygen species and activation of miR-27b expression." Free Radical Biology and Medicine 68: 288-301.

Rastogi, R. P. and R. P. Sinha (2010). "Apoptosis: molecular mechanisms and pathogenicity."

Rasul Suleria, H. A., M. Sadiq Butt, F. Muhammad Anjum, F. Saeed, R. Batool and A. Nisar Ahmad (2012). "Aqueous garlic extract and its phytochemical profile; special reference to antioxidant status." Int J Food Sci Nutr 63(4): 431-439.

Ribeiro, D. A., D. M. Salvadori and M. E. Marques (2005). "Abnormal expression of bcl-2 and bax in rat tongue mucosa during the development of squamous cell carcinoma induced by 4-nitroquinoline 1-oxide." International journal of experimental pathology 86(6): 375-382.

Rice-Evans, C. A., N. J. Miller and G. Paganga (1996). "Structure-antioxidant activity relationships of flavonoids and phenolic acids." Free Radical Biology and Medicine 20(7): 933-956.

Roleira, F. M. F., E. J. Tavares-da-Silva, C. L. Varela, S. C. Costa, T. Silva, J. Garrido and F. Borges (2015). "Plant derived and dietary phenolic antioxidants: Anticancer properties." Food Chemistry 183: 235-258.

Rotruck, J. T., A. L. Pope, H. Ganther, A. Swanson, D. G. Hafeman and W. Hoekstra (1973). "Selenium: biochemical role as a component of glutathione peroxidase." Science 179(4073): 588-590.

Ruggeri, B. A., F. Camp and S. Miknyoczki (2014). "Animal models of disease: preclinical animal models of cancer and their applications and utility in drug discovery." Biochemical pharmacology 87(1): 150-161.

Ryu, M. J. and H. S. Chung (2015). "[10]-Gingerol induces mitochondrial apoptosis through activation of MAPK pathway in HCT116 human colon cancer cells." In Vitro Cellular & Developmental Biology - Animal 51(1): 92-101.

Saif, M. W., I. A. Siddiqui and M. A. Sohail (2009). "Management of ascites due to gastrointestinal malignancy." Annals of Saudi medicine 29(5): 369.

Salinas, J., T. Georgiev, J. A. González-Sánchez, E. López-Ruiz and J. A. Rodríguez-Montes (2014). "Gastric necrosis: A late complication of nissen fundoplication." World journal of gastrointestinal surgery 6(9): 183.

Salzman, R., K. Kankova, L. Pacal, J. Tomandl, Z. Horakova and R. Kostrica (2007). "Increased activity of superoxide dismutase in advanced stages of head and neck squamous cell carcinoma with locoregional metastases." Neoplasma 54(4): 321-325.

Sanner, M. F. (1999). "Python: a programming language for software integration and development." J Mol Graph Model 17(1): 57-61.

Sano, T. and T. Aiko (2011). "New Japanese classifications and treatment guidelines for gastric cancer: revision concepts and major revised points." Gastric cancer 14(2): 97.

Santoro, E. (2005). "The history of gastric cancer: legends and chronicles." Gastric Cancer 8(2): 71-74.

Sapolsky, A. I., R. D. Altman, J. F. Woessner and D. S. Howell (1973). "The action of cathepsin D in human articular cartilage on proteoglycans." The Journal of clinical investigation 52(3): 624-633.

Sarkar, F. H. and Y. Li (2008). "NF-kappaB: a potential target for cancer chemoprevention and therapy." Frontiers in bioscience: a journal and virtual library 13: 2950-2959.

Sauer, B. (1987). "Functional expression of the cre-lox site-specific recombination system in the yeast Saccharomyces cerevisiae." Molecular and cellular biology 7(6): 2087-2096.

Sawyers, C. (2004). "Targeted cancer therapy." Nature 432(7015): 294.

Schlake, T. and J. Bode (1994). "Use of mutated FLP recognition target (FRT) sites for the exchange of expression cassettes at defined chromosomal loci." Biochemistry 33(43): 12746-12751.

Sen, C. K. (2001). "Antioxidants in exercise nutrition." Sports Medicine 31(13): 891-908.

Seto, M., K. Honma and M. Nakagawa (2010). "Diversity of genome profiles in malignant lymphoma." Cancer science 101(3): 573-578.

Shabir, G. A. (2003). "Validation of high-performance liquid chromatography methods for pharmaceutical analysis: Understanding the differences and similarities between validation requirements of the US Food and Drug Administration, the US Pharmacopeia and the International Conference on Harmonization." Journal of chromatography A **987**(1-2): 57-66.

Shanmugam, K. R., K. Mallikarjuna, N. Kesireddy and K. Sathyavelu Reddy (2011). "Neuroprotective effect of ginger on anti-oxidant enzymes in streptozotocin-induced diabetic rats." Food and Chemical Toxicology **49**(4): 893-897.

Shao, S. L., W. W. Zhang and F. Y. Li (2012). Apoptosis of human gastric cancer cell Line SGC-7901 induced by allicin. Advanced Materials Research, Trans Tech Publ.

Sharma, A. and V. Radhakrishnan (2011). "Gastric cancer in India." Indian J Med Paediatr Oncol **32**(1): 12-16.

Sharma, G., J. Ardila-Gatas, M. Boules, M. Davis, J. Villamere, J. Rodriguez, S. A. Brethauer, J. Ponsky and M. Kroh (2016). "Upper gastrointestinal endoscopy is safe and feasible in the early postoperative period after Roux-en-Y gastric bypass." Surgery **160**(4): 885-891.

Sharpless, N. E. and R. A. DePinho (2006). "Model organisms: The mighty mouse: genetically engineered mouse models in cancer drug development." Nature reviews Drug discovery **5**(9): 741.

Shaw, M. J., N. J. Talley, T. J. Beebe, T. Rockwood, R. Carlsson, S. Adlis, A. M. Fendrick, R. Jones, J. Dent and P. Bytzer (2001). "Initial validation of a diagnostic questionnaire for gastroesophageal reflux disease." The American journal of gastroenterology **96**(1): 52-57.

Sheen, L.-Y., H.-W. Chen, Y.-L. Kung, C.-T. Liu and C.-K. Lii (1999). "Effects of Garlic Oil and Its Organosulfur Compounds on the Activities of Hepatic Drug-Metabolizing and Antioxidant Enzymes in Rats Fed High- and Low-Fat Diets." Nutrition and Cancer **35**(2): 160-166.

Shi, Q.-Y. and V. Schlegel (2012). "Green tea as an agricultural based health promoting food: the past five to ten years." Agriculture **2**(4): 393-413.

Shikata, K., Y. Kiyohara, M. Kubo, K. Yonemoto, T. Ninomiya, T. Shirota, Y. Tanizaki, K. Tanaka, Y. Oishi and T. Matsumoto (2006). "A prospective study of dietary salt intake and gastric cancer incidence in a defined Japanese population: the Hisayama study." International journal of cancer **119**(1): 196-201.

Shukla, Y. and M. Singh (2007). "Cancer preventive properties of ginger: a brief review." Food and chemical toxicology **45**(5): 683-690.

Singletary, K. W., M. J. Stansbury, M. Giusti, R. B. Van Breemen, M. Wallig and A. Rimando (2003). "Inhibition of rat mammary tumorigenesis by concord grape juice constituents." Journal of agricultural and food chemistry **51**(25): 7280-7286.

Sinha, A. K. (1972). "Colorimetric assay of catalase." Analytical biochemistry **47**(2): 389-394.

Sintara, K., D. Thong-Ngam, S. Patumraj and N. Klaikeaw (2012). "Curcumin attenuates gastric cancer induced by N-methyl-N-nitrosourea and saturated sodium chloride in rats." BioMed Research International **2012**.

Sparnins, V. L., G. Barany and L. W. Wattenberg (1988). "Effects of organosulfur compounds from garlic and onions on benzo [a] pyrene-induced neoplasia and glutathione S-transferase activity in the mouse." Carcinogenesis 9(1): 131-134.

Srinivasan, K. (2014). "Antioxidant potential of spices and their active constituents." Critical reviews in food science and nutrition 54(3): 352-372.

Srinivasan, K. (2017). "Antimutagenic and cancer preventive potential of culinary spices and their bioactive compounds." PharmaNutrition 5(3): 89-102.

Staal, G. E., J. Visser and C. Veeger (1969). "Purification and properties of glutathione reductase of human erythrocytes." Biochimica et Biophysica Acta (BBA)-Enzymology 185(1): 39-48.

Stewart, T. A., P. K. Pattengale and P. Leder (1984). "Spontaneous mammary adenocarcinomas in transgenic mice that carry and express MTV/myc fusion genes." Cell 38(3): 627-637.

Sundaresan, S. and P. Subramanian (2003). "S-allylcysteine inhibits circulatory lipid peroxidation and promotes antioxidants in N-nitrosodiethylamine-induced carcinogenesis." Polish journal of pharmacology 55(1): 37-42.

Sung, N., K. Choi, E. Park, K. Park, S. Lee, A. Lee, I. Choi, K. Jung, Y. Won and H. Shin (2007). "Smoking, alcohol and gastric cancer risk in Korean men: the National Health Insurance Corporation Study." British Journal of Cancer 97(5): 700-704.

Surh, Y.-J., K.-S. Chun, H.-H. Cha, S. S. Han, Y.-S. Keum, K.-K. Park and S. S. Lee (2001). "Molecular mechanisms underlying chemopreventive activities of anti-inflammatory phytochemicals: down-regulation of COX-2 and iNOS through suppression of NF-κB activation." Mutation Research/Fundamental and Molecular Mechanisms of Mutagenesis 480: 243-268.

Taha, M. M., A. B. Abdul, R. Abdullah, T. A. Ibrahim, S. I. Abdelwahab and S. Mohan (2010). "Potential chemoprevention of diethylnitrosamine-initiated and 2-acetylaminofluorene-promoted hepatocarcinogenesis by zerumbone from the rhizomes of the subtropical ginger (Zingiber zerumbet)." Chem Biol Interact 186(3): 295-305.

Talas, Z. S., I. Ozdemir, I. Yilmaz and Y. Gok (2009). "Antioxidative effects of novel synthetic organoselenium compound in rat lung and kidney." Ecotoxicology and environmental safety 72(3): 916-921.

Talley, N. J., M. Verlinden and M. Jones (2001). "Can symptoms discriminate among those with delayed or normal gastric emptying in dysmotility-like dyspepsia?" The American journal of gastroenterology 96(5): 1422-1428.

Tao, J., Y. Li, S. Li and H.-B. Li (2018). "Plant foods for the prevention and management of colon cancer." Journal of Functional Foods 42: 95-110.

Teoh-Fitzgerald, M. L., M. P. Fitzgerald, T. J. Jensen, B. W. Futscher and F. E. Domann (2012). "Genetic and epigenetic inactivation of extracellular superoxide dismutase promotes an invasive phenotype in human lung cancer by disrupting ECM homeostasis." Mol Cancer Res **10**(1): 40-51.

Thirunavukkarasu, C. and D. Sakthisekaran (2001). "Effect of selenium on N-nitrosodiethylamine-induced multistage hepatocarcinogenesis with reference to lipid peroxidation and enzymic antioxidants." Cell biochemistry and function **19**(1): 27-35.

Thomas, K. R. and M. R. Capecchi (1987). "Site-directed mutagenesis by gene targeting in mouse embryo-derived stem cells." Cell **51**(3): 503-512.

Thompson, C. B. (1995). "Apoptosis in the pathogenesis and treatment of disease." Science **267**(5203): 1456-1462.

Tjendraputra, E., V. H. Tran, D. Liu-Brennan, B. D. Roufogalis and C. C. Duke (2001). "Effect of ginger constituents and synthetic analogues on cyclooxygenase-2 enzyme in intact cells." Bioorganic chemistry **29**(3): 156-163.

Towbin, H., T. Staehelin and J. Gordon (1979). "Electrophoretic transfer of proteins from polyacrylamide gels to nitrocellulose sheets: procedure and some applications." Proceedings of the National Academy of Sciences **76**(9): 4350-4354.

Trachootham, D., W. Lu, M. A. Ogasawara, N. R.-D. Valle and P. Huang (2008). "Redox regulation of cell survival." Antioxidants & redox signaling **10**(8): 1343-1374.

Traverso, N., R. Ricciarelli, M. Nitti, B. Marengo, A. L. Furfaro, M. A. Pronzato, U. M. Marinari and C. Domenicotti (2013). "Role of glutathione in cancer progression and chemoresistance." Oxidative medicine and cellular longevity **2013**.

Tsubura, A., Y. C. Lai, M. Kuwata, N. Uehara and K. Yoshizawa (2011). "Anticancer effects of garlic and garlic-derived compounds for breast cancer control." Anticancer Agents Med Chem **11**(3): 249-253.

Tsukamoto, H., T. Mizoshita, T. Katano, N. Hayashi, K. Ozeki, M. Ebi, T. Shimura, Y. Mori, S. Tanida and H. Kataoka (2015). "Preventive effect of rebamipide on N-methyl-N'-nitro-N-nitrosoguanidine-induced gastric carcinogenesis in rats." Experimental and Toxicologic Pathology **67**(3): 271-277.

Tuffaha, M. S., H. Guski and G. Kristiansen (2018). Recommendations for the Utility of Immunohistochemistry in Tumor Diagnosis. Immunohistochemistry in Tumor Diagnostics, Springer: 257-258.

Uemura, N., S. Okamoto, S. Yamamoto, N. Matsumura, S. Yamaguchi, M. Yamakido, K. Taniyama, N. Sasaki and R. J. Schlemper (2001). "Helicobacter pylori infection and the development of gastric cancer." New England Journal of Medicine **345**(11): 784-789.

Valko, M., D. Leibfritz, J. Moncol, M. T. Cronin, M. Mazur and J. Telser (2007). "Free radicals and antioxidants in normal physiological functions and human disease." The international journal of biochemistry & cell biology **39**(1): 44-84.

van Poppel, G. and H. van den Berg (1997). "Vitamins and cancer." Cancer letters **114**(1): 195-202.

van Poppel, G., D. T. Verhoeven, H. Verhagen and R. A. Goldbohm (1999). Brassica vegetables and cancer prevention. Advances in Nutrition and Cancer 2, Springer: 159-168.

Venkatesh, S., M. Deecaraman, R. Kumar, M. Shamsi and R. Dada (2009). "Role of reactive oxygen species in the pathogenesis of mitochondrial DNA (mtDNA) mutations in male infertility." Indian Journal of Medical Research 129(2).

Verpoorte, R., Y. H. Choi and H. K. Kim (2005). "Ethnopharmacology and systems biology: a perfect holistic match." Journal of Ethnopharmacology 100(1-2): 53-56.

Voskoglou-Nomikos, T., J. L. Pater and L. Seymour (2003). "Clinical predictive value of the in vitro cell line, human xenograft, and mouse allograft preclinical cancer models." Clinical Cancer Research 9(11): 4227-4239.

Wagner, H. and G. Ulrich-Merzenich (2009). "Synergy research: approaching a new generation of phytopharmaceuticals." Phytomedicine 16(2-3): 97-110.

Waldum, H. L., L. Sagatun and P. Mjønes (2017). "Gastrin and gastric cancer." Frontiers in endocrinology 8: 1.

Wang, H. C., Y. L. Chu, S. C. Hsieh and L. Y. Sheen (2017). "Diallyl trisulfide inhibits cell migration and invasion of human melanoma a375 cells via inhibiting integrin/facal adhesion kinase pathway." Environmental toxicology 32(11): 2352-2359.

Wang, X. (2001). "The expanding role of mitochondria in apoptosis." Genes & development 15(22): 2922-2933.

Wang, X., F. Jiao, Q.-W. Wang, J. Wang, K. Yang, R.-R. Hu, H.-C. Liu, H.-Y. Wang and Y.-S. Wang (2012). "Aged black garlic extract induces inhibition of gastric cancer cell growth in vitro and in vivo." Molecular medicine reports 5(1): 66-72.

Waris, G. and H. Ahsan (2006). "Reactive oxygen species: role in the development of cancer and various chronic conditions." Journal of carcinogenesis 5: 14.

Wu, C. S., M. F. Chen, I. L. Lee and S. Y. Tung (2007). "Predictive role of nuclear factor-kappaB activity in gastric cancer: a promising adjuvant approach with caffeic acid phenethyl ester." J Clin Gastroenterol 41(10): 894-900.

Wu, G., Y.-Z. Fang, S. Yang, J. R. Lupton and N. D. Turner (2004). "Glutathione metabolism and its implications for health." The Journal of nutrition 134(3): 489-492.

Wu, L. and M. de Perrot (2017). "Radio-immunotherapy and chemo-immunotherapy as a novel treatment paradigm in malignant pleural mesothelioma." Translational lung cancer research 6(3): 325.

Yamachika, T., H. Nakanishi, K. i. Inada, T. Tsukamoto, N. Shimizu, K. Kobayashi, S. Fukushima and M. Tatematsu (1998). "N-Methyl-N-nitrosourea concentration-dependent, rather than total intake-dependent, induction of adenocarcinomas in the glandular stomach of BALB/c mice." Cancer Science **89**(4): 385-391.

Yamamoto, M., C. Furihata, T. Ogiu, T. Tsukamoto, K.-i. Inada, K. Hirano and M. Tatematsu (2002). "Independent variation in susceptibilities of six different mouse strains to induction of pepsinogen-altered pyloric glands and gastric tumor intestinalization by N-methyl-N-nitrosourea." Cancer letters **179**(2): 121-132.

Yamamoto, Y. and R. B. Gaynor (2001). "Therapeutic potential of inhibition of the NF-κB pathway in the treatment of inflammation and cancer." The Journal of clinical investigation **107**(2): 135-142.

Yanaka, A., J. W. Fahey, A. Fukumoto, M. Nakayama, S. Inoue, S. Zhang, M. Tauchi, H. Suzuki, I. Hyodo and M. Yamamoto (2009). "Dietary sulforaphane-rich broccoli sprouts reduce colonization and attenuate gastritis in Helicobacter pylori-infected mice and humans." Cancer Prev Res (Phila) **2**(4): 353-360.

Yang, J., B. Chen and Y. Gu (2012). "Pharmacological evaluation of tea polysaccharides with antioxidant activity in gastric cancer mice." Carbohydrate polymers **90**(2): 943-947.

Yonesaka, K., K. Hirotani, H. Kawakami, M. Takeda, H. Kaneda, K. Sakai, I. Okamoto, K. Nishio, P. Jänne and K. Nakagawa (2016). "Anti-HER3 monoclonal antibody patritumab sensitizes refractory non-small cell lung cancer to the epidermal growth factor receptor inhibitor erlotinib." Oncogene **35**(7): 878-886.

Yoshino, K. (2000). "[History of gastric cancer surgery]." Nihon Geka Gakkai Zasshi **101**(12): 855-860.

Youle, R. J. and A. Strasser (2008). "The BCL-2 protein family: opposing activities that mediate cell death." Nature reviews Molecular cell biology **9**(1): 47.

Yu, B. P. (1994). "Cellular defenses against damage from reactive oxygen species." Physiological reviews **74**(1): 139-162.

Yu, Z., T. Zhang, F. Zhou, X. Xiao, X. Ding, H. He, J. Rang, M. Quan, T. Wang and M. Zuo (2015). "Anticancer activity of saponins from Allium chinense against the B16 melanoma and 4T1 breast carcinoma cell." Evidence-Based Complementary and Alternative Medicine **2015**.

Yun, H.-M., J. O. Ban, K.-R. Park, C. K. Lee, H.-S. Jeong, S. B. Han and J. T. Hong (2014). "Potential therapeutic effects of functionally active compounds isolated from garlic." Pharmacology & therapeutics **142**(2): 183-195.

Zhang, F., J.-G. Zhang, J. Qu, Q. Zhang, C. Prasad and Z.-J. Wei (2017). "Assessment of anti-cancerous potential of 6-gingerol (Tongling White Ginger) and its synergy with drugs on human cervical adenocarcinoma cells." Food and Chemical Toxicology **109**: 910-922.

Zhang, X., Y. Zhu, W. Duan, C. Feng and X. He (2015). "Allicin induces apoptosis of the MGC-803 human gastric carcinoma cell line through the p38 mitogen-activated protein kinase/caspase-3 signaling pathway." Molecular medicine reports **11**(4): 2755-2760.

Zhou, Y., W. Zhuang, W. Hu, G. J. Liu, T. X. Wu and X. T. Wu (2011). "Consumption of large amounts of Allium vegetables reduces risk for gastric cancer in a meta-analysis." Gastroenterology **141**(1): 80-89.

Zimmermann, G. R., J. Lehar and C. T. Keith (2007). "Multi-target therapeutics: when the whole is greater than the sum of the parts." Drug discovery today **12**(1-2): 34-42.

Zou, H., R. Yang, J. Hao, J. Wang, C. Sun, S. W. Fesik, J. C. Wu, K. J. Tomaselli and R. C. Armstrong (2003). "Regulation of the Apaf-1/caspase-9 apoptosome by caspase-3 and XIAP." Journal of Biological Chemistry **278**(10): 8091-8098.

Zou, X., J. Liang, J. Sun, X. Hu, L. Lei, D. Wu and L. Liu (2016). "Allicin sensitizes hepatocellular cancer cells to anti-tumor activity of 5-fluorouracil through ROS-mediated mitochondrial pathway." Journal of Pharmacological Sciences **131**(4): 233-240.

# ANNEXURES

# ANNEXURE I

## Ethical Committee Clearance Certificate

**PONDICHERRY UNIVERSITY**
R.V.Nagar, Kalapet, Puducherry- 605014

Dr. A. Hannah Rachel Vasanthi, M.Sc., M.Phil., Ph.D.
Associate Professor, Biotechnology
Member Secretary
Institutional Animal Ethics Committee

Tele: 0413-2654 745
Tele Fax: 0413-2656 742
E.mail.:hrvasanthi@gmail.com

PU/SLS/AH/14th IAEC/2016/4                                    29.03.2016

To
Ms. Debjani P.M.
Ph.D. Scholar
Dept. of Biotechnology
School of Life Sciences
Pondicherry University

Dear Ms. Debjani,

    Please refer to your proposal entitled "Evaluation of Chemopreventive effects of selected Indian spices against chemical induced gastric cancer in male Wistar rats" for consideration and approval of IAEC.

    I wish to inform you that your above said proposal was considered by IAEC, Pondicherry University in its 14th meeting held on 23.03.2016. The detail of the decision taken is quoted below.

Thanking you,

Yours Sincerely,

(A. Hannah Rachel Vasanthi)
**MEMBER SECRETARY**
IAEC
School of Life Sciences
Pondicherry University
Puducherry-14

---

**Recommendations of Institutional Animal Ethics Committee**

**Ms. Debjani P. Mansingh** Ph.D Scholar, Department of Biotechnology, working under the supervision of Dr. A. Hannah Rachel Vasanthi submitted a project entitled "Evaluation of Chemopreventive effects of selected Indian spices against chemical induced gastric cancer in male Wistar rats" and 90 male Wistar albino rats were requested.

    The committee approved only 90 male Wistar albino rats for the Ph.D work and cautioned the safe use and disposal of carcinogenic agent in the animal house.

# ANNEXURE II

## List of Publications

1. **Debjani P. Mansingh,** Nibedita Dalpati, Veeresh Kumar Sali and Hannah R. Vasanthi Alliin the precursor of Allicin in garlic extract mitigates proliferation of gastric adenocarcinoma cells by modulating apoptosis. *Pharmacognosy Magazine* **2018** (In Press) **(IF-1.09)**

2. Veeresh Kumar Sali, **Debjani P. Mansingh** and Hannah R. Vasanthi. Relative apoptotic potential and specific G1 arrest of stigmasterol and cinnamic acid isolated from the brown algae *Padina gymnospora* in HeLa and A549 cells. *Med. Chem. Commun.,* **2016**, *7*, 1429-1435. **(IF-2.31)**

3. Mabel Parimala, **Debjani P. Mansingh,** Hannah R Vasanthi, Francis Gricilda Shoba. *Nymphaea nouchali* Burm. hydroalcoholic seed extract increases glucose consumption in 3T3-L1 adipocytes through activation of peroxisome proliferator-activated receptor gamma and insulin sensitization. *J. Adv. Pharm Technol Res.* **2015** Oct-Dec; *6*(4): 183–189.

**ANNEXURE-III**

**Fellowship**

Basic Scientific Research Fellowship (BSR-UGC 2012-2017) from University Grants Commission (UGC), India.

ANNEXURE-IV

## Contributions in Conferences/Seminars

1. **Debjani Payoswini Mansingh** participated in the National Workshop and Industry-Academia Interaction Meet on Drugs and Pharmaceuticals-Research and Development $12^{th}$-$13^{th}$ April, 2013. Conducted by Department of Biotechnology, School of Life Sciences, Pondicherry University, Puducherry.

2. **Debjani Payoswini Mansingh** presented a paper on **"Influence of Ginger and Garlic Extract and its Major Bioactive Constituents on Gastric Adenocarcinoma Cells"** in the International conference on Recent Advances in Research and Treatment of Human diseases and $4^{th}$ annual meeting of Indian academy of biomedical sciences at Indian Institute of Chemical Technology $9^{th}$-$11^{th}$ January 2015.

3. **Debjani Payoswini Mansingh** presented a research work on **"Influence of Ginger and its Major Bioactive Molecule in AGS Cells"** in the $36^{th}$ Annual conference of Indian Association of Biomedical Scientists on "Translational Sciences: Bridging Ancient and Modern Biomedicine" Organized by Dept of Biotechnology, Pondicherry University $17^{th}$ to $20^{th}$ December 2015.

4. **Debjani Payoswini Mansingh** participated in the National Workshop on Flow cytometry conducted by Department of Biotechnology, Sri Ramachandra University, $15^{th}$-$18^{th}$ October 2016.

5. **Debjani Payoswini Mansingh** presented a research work on **"Alliin in Garlic Modulates Inflammation in Gastric Adenocarcinoma (AGS) Cells"** in the First International Conference on "Nutraceuticals and Chronic Diseases. Organized by Indian Institute of Technology $20^{th}$-$24^{th}$ October 2016.

# Alliin the Precursor of Allicin in Garlic Extract Mitigates Proliferation of Gastric Adenocarcinoma Cells by Modulating Apoptosis

Debjani P. Mansingh, Nibedita Dalpati, Veeresh Kumar Sali, A. Hannah Rachel Vasanthi[1]

Department of Biotechnology, Natural Products Research Laboratory, School of Life Sciences, Pondicherry University, Pondicherry University, Puducherry, India

Submitted: 02-08-2017  Revised: 08-09-2017  Published: ???

## ABSTRACT

**Background:** Garlic, a common spice used since time immemorial for various purposes, is considered a potential functional food as it exhibits cardioprotection to chemoprevention properties due to the presence of organosulfur constituents in each garlic pod. Alliin is not widely studied for its bioactivity as it is an unstable compound which is converted to allicin on mechanical and chemical degradation. **Objective:** Hence, in the present study, the influence of alliin on gastric adenocarcinoma (AGS) cells and normal intestinal cells (INT-407) would be tested for its potent antiproliferative effect and mechanism of action. **Materials and Methods:** The quantity of alliin in fresh and dried garlic extract was measured by high-performance liquid chromatography to corroborate the cytotoxicity activity identified by 3-(4,5-dimethylthiazol-2-yl)-2,5-diphenyl tetrazolium bromide assay and acridine orange/ethidium bromide staining. Further, to identify the mechanism of action, DNA fragmentation assay, annexin V Assay, and flow cytometry analysis of apoptosis followed by expression of apoptotic proteins such as Bax, Bcl-2, and cytochrome-C by Western blot was done. **Results:** It was identified that alliin inhibited proliferation of gastric carcinoma cells by decreasing the cell viability but not in the normal intestinal cells. The level of apoptosis was modulated by reactive oxygen species generation and decrease in mitochondrial membrane potential mediated by deregulation of Bax/Bcl-2 level at protein level leading to upregulation of Cytochrome C. **Conclusion:** It is impressive to note that alliin content was high in fresh aqueous extract compared to that of dried garlic extract which concludes that the use of garlic from time immemorial is a worthy functional food in its fresh form to combat cancer cells. However, *in-vivo* studies are warranted.
**Key words:** Alliin, apoptosis, DNA fragmentation, gastric adenocarcinoma, gastric cancer, reactive oxygen species

### SUMMARY

* Alliin a precursor of allicin in garlic extract exhibits anti-proliferative potential in gastric adenocarcinoma cells
* The bioactivity is mediated by apoptosis which was modulated by reactive oxygen species generation, alteration of membrane potential through extrinsic and intrinsic pathway
* However, this was not noticed in normal intestinal cells proving it to be a phytonutrient of functional properties used from ancient times.

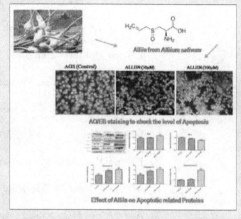

**Abbreviations used:** AGS-Gastric adenocarcinoma; ROS-Reactive oxygen species; MMP-Mitochondrial membrane potential; TBS- Tris buffered saline.

**Correspondence:**
Dr. A. Hannah Rachel Vasanthi,
Department of Biotechnology,
Pondicherry University, Puducherry - 605 014, India.
E-mail: hrvasanthi@gmail.com
DOI: 10.4103/pm.pm_342_17

**Access this article online**
Website: www.phcog.com
Quick Response Code:

## INTRODUCTION

Cancers account for around 8.2 million deaths worldwide making it the major reason for death.[1] Although the symptoms and signs of stomach cancer are observed only in the advanced stage, stomach cancer ranks the second-most prevalent cancer among males and third-most among females both globally and in Asia.[2] More than 70% of stomach cancer cases occur in developing countries which accounts for a 5-year survival rate of <30% with half the world's total cases occurring in Eastern Asia as compared to 20% in developing countries.[2-4] Among the different types of stomach cancers, gastric cancers are more prevalent since a wide range of factors such as diet, lifestyle, age, and genetic factors influence the susceptibility to gastric cancers. Consumption of natural foods which includes fruits, vegetables, spices, nuts, and beverages such as wine and tea has influenced the prevention and management of cancers due to the presence of specific phytochemicals which attenuates pathologies

This is an open access article distributed under the terms of the Creative Commons Attribution-NonCommercial-ShareAlike 3.0 License, which allows others to remix, tweak, and build upon the work non-commercially, as long as the author is credited and the new creations are licensed under the identical terms.

For reprints contact: reprints@medknow.com

**Cite this article as:** Mansingh DP, Dalpati N, Sali VK, Vasanthi HR. Alliin the precursor of allicin in garlic extract mitigates proliferation of gastric adenocarcinoma cells by modulating apoptosis. Phcog Mag 2018;XX:XX-XX.

# MedChemComm

## RESEARCH ARTICLE

Cite this: DOI: 10.1039/c6md00178e

# Relative apoptotic potential and specific G1 arrest of stigmasterol and cinnamic acid isolated from the brown algae *Padina gymnospora* in HeLa and A549 cells†

Veeresh Kumar Sali, Debjani P. Mansingh and Hannah R. Vasanthi*

This study aimed to isolate, chemically characterize and determine the apoptotic potential of small molecules from the methanol extract of the marine brown algae *Padina gymnospora* collected from the Mandapam coast. The data obtained showed that a) by FT-NMR spectral results and comparison with the SDBS database, compound 1 was identified to be stigmasterol (SS) and compound 2 was identified as cinnamic acid (CA). b) The growth inhibitory activities in terms of $IC_{50}$ value of SS treated A549 and HeLa cells are 10.36 μM and 12.21 μM, respectively, and those of CA are 50.18 μM and 24.81 μM, respectively at 24 h. c) The influence of SS and CA induced apoptosis was morphologically confirmed using a fluorescence microscope by AO/EB dual staining. d) The cell cycle analysis clearly demonstrates that CA treated HeLa cell growth was significantly arrested at the G1 phase. In the case of A549 cells, CA did not show any significant growth arrest. CA induced an accumulation of cells in G1 phase at the highest concentration, suggesting a block in the transition from G1 to S phase. e) Results from docking studies suggest that SS and CA bind the p53-binding pocket of MDM2, thereby displacing p53, which in turn sensitizes cancer cells to these anticancer agents.

Received 28th March 2016,
Accepted 28th April 2016

DOI: 10.1039/c6md00178e

www.rsc.org/medchemcomm

## Introduction

Apoptosis, the process of programmed cell death, is critically important during various developmental processes and aging and exhibits a homeostatic mechanism to maintain cell population in tissues.[1] Apoptosis also occurs to eliminate activated or auto-aggressive immune cells either during maturation in the central lymphoid organs (bone marrow and thymus) or in peripheral tissues as a defence mechanism, or when cells are damaged by disease or noxious agents.[2] Abnormalities in cell death regulation can be a significant component of several diseases, such as ischemic damage, autoimmune diseases and many types of cancer.[3] Cancer is the prime example of a disease status where the normal mechanisms of cell cycle regulation are dysfunctional, with overproliferation of cells and/ or decreased removal of cells.[4] Tumor cells use a variety of molecular mechanisms to suppress apoptosis.[5] A crucial mechanism includes the inactivation of the p53 pathway. Hence, identifying a bioactive molecule from natural products or chemically synthesizing and further identifying its molecular mechanism of action is a worthwhile effort.

In recent times, as part of the Drugs from the Sea programme in several parts of the world, several bioactive compounds have been isolated and characterized from marine organisms. However, despite recent progress in the area of marine chemistry, the marine flora of the Indian Ocean have been less explored, which motivated us to investigate the chemical constituents of these marine flora and study their role in apoptosis in cancer cells. *Padina gymnospora*, a brown alga belonging to the family Dictyoaceae, is abundant in the southeast coast of India. As part of our ongoing quest for anticancer compounds from the seaweeds of the Gulf of Mannar, we have reported some natural compounds obtained from the methanol extract of this alga. In the present study, cinnamic acid and stigmasterol were isolated and characterized using FT-NMR (Fourier Transform Nuclear Magnetic Resonance), and the chemical shift values were compared with the SDBS Database. Moreover, the cytotoxic activities of the isolated compounds on lung adeno carcinoma cells (A549) and cervical cancer cells (HeLa) were studied to confirm their potential as apoptotic agents. The study gives insights on the efficacy of the sterol moiety isolated from the marine algae in comparison with cinnamic acid, a non sterol compound, as an anticancer agent. Further, the mechanism by which these molecules exhibit tumor suppression mediated by p53 was confirmed by *in silico* docking analysis.

*Department of Biotechnology, School of Life Sciences, Pondicherry University, Puducherry – 605014, India. E-mail: hrvasanthi@gmail.com*
† Authors declare no competing interests.

# PROPHYLACTIC AND THERAPEUTIC ACTIVITY OF GINGER AND GARLIC IN EXPERIMENTALLY INDUCED GASTRIC CANCER

*A thesis submitted in partial fulfillment of the requirement for the award of the degree of*

DOCTOR OF PHILOSOPHY

In

BIOTECHNOLOGY

By

**DEBJANI PAYOSWINI MANSINGH**
Reg Id: R 29237

*Under the guidance of*

**Prof. A. HANNAH RACHEL VASANTHI**
DEPARTMENT OF BIOTECHNOLOGY
SCHOOL OF LIFE SCIENCE

**PONDICHERRY UNIVERSITY
PUDUCHERRY - 605014
INDIA**

April 2018

# CHAPTER 5

## Summary, Conclusion and Recommendation

# CHAPTER 5

## 5.1 Summary

The uncontrolled growth of cancerous cells known as metastasis is a long term multifaceted dynamic process which leads to the development of cancer. Natural products are key agents used for preventing and managing devastating diseases like cancer encountered by mankind. More specifically, they exhibit anticancer potential owing to the existence of bioactive compounds in them such as flavonoids, anthocyanins, lignins, sterols, etc. Likewise, micronutrients in natural product derived diet such as vitamins, trace elements and antioxidants play a pivotal role in reducing cell damage and may act synergistically to enhance several protective mechanisms against carcinogenesis. Researchers have demonstrated that several dietary components of natural origin possess the capacity to prevent and manage cancer. The possible mechanisms include increased detoxification of carcinogens, cell differentiation, maintenance of DNA repair, decrease in cell proliferation and increased apoptosis/autophagy of cancer cells mediated by antioxidant effects and alteration in mitochondrial membrane potential, ER stress etc. Unlike other diseases, cancer exhibits an uncanny ability to remain incognizant to a wide range of treatment approaches. This quality could be attributed to many reasons behind the cause and management of cancer. One such complicated cancer type owing to the various causative agents is gastric cancer affecting more than one million people throughout the world. Further, the identification of the disease at an early stage is farfetched as there are no early diagnostic biomarkers identified for gastric cancer. To add on, treatment of gastric cancer involves a heavy dose of strong drugs which have severe side effects. The repercussions of treatment include early mortality along with organ failure. Hence, identifying functional drugs/foods with fewer side effects which can exhibit both prophylactic and therapeutic effect is worth identifying.

Drug discovery and development through rigorous R&D is a tedious, time and resource driven process. Hence, in the present study two commonly used spices ginger and garlic and its phytoconstituents which also possess medicinal property was selected to reveal its anticancer potential both individually and in combination by *in silico*, *in vitro* and *in vivo* studies.

Computer facilitated approaches such as docking, pharmacophore modelling and virtual screening would potentially save time and resource in drug discovery and development, directing to more promising novel agents and expediting the process. Drug discovery is anticipated to be expedited through the combined use of experimentation and bioinformatics. Inflammation and apoptosis are two major hallmarks of cancer pathology and identifying specific targets to maneuver these pathologies would be ideal to manage the deadly disease. Therefore, to find out the best bioactive lead present in ginger and garlic to combat cancer, the *in-silico* docking analysis of different phytocompounds of ginger ([6]-Gingerol, [10]-Gingerol, [8]-Shogal, Zingerone) and garlic (Alliin, Allicin, Diallydisulphide, *S*-allyl cysteine) with pro-inflammatory markers and apoptotic markers was studied. [6]-Gingerol and Alliin interact strongly with NFkB and COX-2. Likewise, they showed strong binding energy with the apoptotic markers Bax and Bcl2 in comparison to the other molecules of ginger and garlic. Hence, these bioactive leads ([6]-Gingerol and Alliin) were chosen for all *in-vitro* molecular mechanistic studies.

After identifying that the two compounds are potent by *in silico* analysis, [6]-Gingerol, the major phytocompound from Ginger as well as Alliin, the abundant phytoconstituent in Garlic were quantified by HPLC in both fresh and dried forms. It was found out that [6]-

Gingerol content in the aqueous extract of fresh ginger was more in comparison to dried ginger extract. Similarly, Alliin content in the aqueous extract of fresh garlic was observed to be more than the dried garlic extracts. Since cancer pathogenesis involves the generation of many free radicals due to oxidative stress, we found it worth studying the role of these extracts as well as their pure compounds as free radical scavengers by some reliable and reproducible methods which includes 2,2-diphenyl-1-picrylhydrazyl (DPPH), Lipid Peroxidation (LPO) inhibition assay and Ferric reducing antioxidant potential assay (FRAP). These assays confirm the potent antioxidant and free scavenging potential of fresh ginger and garlic extracts in comparison to their dried counterparts.

Subsequently, anticancer efficacy of [6]-Gingerol and Alliin was then assessed using AGS cell lines. Cell viability by MTT assay was performed to check the cytotoxic potential of both [6]-Gingerol and Alliin against AGS cells which showed potent cytotoxic effect at an $IC_{50}$ value of 50 μM (Alliin) and 100 μM ([6]-Gingerol). It is interesting to note that when both compounds were tested against INT-407 normal intestinal cell line, they neither induced proliferation nor inhibited the cell growth. Further to check the morphological features of apoptosis mediated by [6]-Gingerol and Alliin, AO/EB staining was performed which was in accordance with the MTT results and proved that both compounds induced apoptosis. Phosphatidylserine externalization by the Annexin-V assay revealed a higher percentage of early apoptotic cells i.e. 56.4% in the case of Alliin and 37.4% in [6]-Gingerol treated cells by flow cytometric analysis. The percentage of cells actively undergoing early apoptosis as well as late apoptosis by [6]-Gingerol and Alliin showed that these phytocompounds markedly influences apoptosis. Further in order to determine whether suppression of cell proliferation by the test compounds inhibit cell cycle progression, AGS cells treated with $IC_{50}$ dose of both the compounds individually for 24 h was checked for DNA fluorescence in propidium iodide-stained cells by flow cytometer. The results confirmed that [6]-Gingerol caused a buildup of cells in the G2/M phase and cell death in the cancer cells while Alliin caused an inflation of S phase cells and a corresponding reduction of cells in the G2/M phase.

Subsequently to unravel the possible mode of action of the test molecules, AGS cells were monitored by staining with 2, 7-dichlorofluorescein diacetate (DCFH-DA) to identify the presence of ROS. Present investigation confirmed noticeable elevation of intracellular ROS induced by the two phytocompounds ([6]-Gingerol and Alliin) in AGS cells compared to the control cells treated with DMSO. Electron and proton transport through the inner membrane of the mitochondria is liable for cellular ROS generation. Accordingly, the mitochondrial membrane potential is altered by mediating apoptosis. Herein, MMP examined by flow cytometric analysis showed that compared to control, [6]-Gingerol and Alliin individually caused a significant loss of MMP after 24 h of treatment. It was evinced that a loss of MMP may be correlated to the production of ROS in AGS cells upon treatment confirmed by DCFDA staining.

The exact mechanistic pathway in mediating apoptosis of AGS cells induced by Alliin and [6]-Gingerol individually was found worth studying. The results of the immunoblot revealed that the level of Cytochrome c in cytosol was enhanced in AGS cells after treating with Alliin (50 µM and 100 µM) and [6]-Gingerol (100 µM and 250 µM) for 24 h. It suggests that Alliin and [6]-Gingerol improved the level of cytochrome c in cytosol which ultimately activates the caspase-dependent and caspase-independent apoptosis pathway. In this study, activation of caspase-9 and caspase-3 also indicates the unalterable or completing stage of apoptosis. Simultaneously, the level of the anti-apoptotic protein Bcl2 and the proapoptotic protein Bax were determined to characterize the mitochondria mediated apoptosis induced by Alliin and [6]-Gingerol. Immunoblots exhibited downregulation of Bcl2 and the upregulation of Bax. It implied that apoptosis of AGS cells by Alliin and [6]-gingerol was mediated by alteration in the level of Pro and anti-apoptotic proteins of Bcl2 family.

Identifying if there exists any combination effect of the phytoconstituents and the extracts of ginger and garlic was worthful. Hence, in this study we performed drug interaction studies to check existence of different combination effect between [6]-Gingerol and Alliin as well as between individual fresh ginger and fresh garlic extracts. In this context, we found out the existence of a moderate antagonism in between [6]-Gingerol and Alliin. Not surprising aqueous extract of both fresh ginger and fresh garlic exhibited synergetic effect which prompted us to confirm the combined synergetic effect of ginger and garlic extract on MNU-induced gastric cancer in experimental animals.

MNU (100 mg/kg b.w.) in citrate buffer, pH-4.5 along with 5% NaCl induction was standardized in albino Wistar rats via intragastric route initially for a period of 8 weeks and then continued till 16 weeks to check the extent of carcinogenicity in male albino Wistar rats. This chemically induced model mimic's gastric cancer than any other model which was evidenced by the reduction in body weight, water intake as well as feed intake in cancer control animals. Oral treatment of individual garlic and ginger extract as well as the combination of both the extracts were administered to rats to prove the therapeutic efficacy on gastric cancer. The increase in body weight as well as feed intake in drug treated rats is noticeable to prove its efficacy. Gastrin, a specific biomarker of gastric carcinogenesis is elevated in MNU induced gastric cancer rats at two time periods (16 weeks and 24 weeks). However, the significant decrease to 4 folds by ginger, garlic extract and their combination is possibly due to the bioactive ingredients present in it which probably suppress the acute and chronic inflammation caused due to MNU-induced gastric carcinogenesis. Enzymes such as alkaline phosphatase (ALP), Glutamyl transferase (γ-GT) and lactate dehydrogenase (LDH) are considered as diagnostic markers for normal liver functioning. Immunological, metabolic or any other insult to the tissues and organs causes elevation of these enzymes in blood of cancer-induced animals. A significant increase of ALP and LDH activity in serum of cancer induced rats is possibly because of damage of the gastrointestinal tissue. Ginger, garlic extract and their combination treated rats exhibited declined ALP and LDH activity possibly due to the protective effect. The synergetic effect of both the ginger and garlic extract was proved for their prophylactic and therapeutic efficacy. A decrease in γ-GT activity was also observed in serum of cancer control rats which clearly shows that γ-GT is independently associated with risk of cancer specific to the liver and not to stomach cancer.

Oxidative stress associated with increased levels of LPO and other thiobarbituric acid reactive substances are linked to cancer progression. An increased lipid peroxidation level in gastric tissues of cancer control group was observed which confirms involvement of oxidative stress in MNU-induced gastric cancer. A significant reduction in LPO levels of ginger extract, garlic extract and their combination extract administered rats could be due to the intake of bioactive nutrients that are believed to act as scavengers of superoxide anions and hydroxyl radicals. Endogenous antioxidants such as catalase, superoxide dismutase (SOD), glutathione peroxidase (GPx), glutathione S-transferase (GST), glutathione reductase (GR) and reduced glutathione (GSH) are labeled as first line defense against noxious free radicals like superoxide and hydrogen peroxides in cellular tissues. The present study showed a significant reduction in SOD, catalase, GST, GPx and GR activity in both stomach and liver tissue of cancer control rats which may be due to enhanced utilization for scavenging lipid peroxides as well as sequestration by tumor cells. It is interesting to note that ginger extract, garlic extract and their combination treated rats elevated the GST, GPx and GR activity in gastric cancer induced rats which proved the prophylactic and therapeutic efficacy of ginger and garlic extract. Reduced glutathione is an important non-protein thiol which belongs to redox cycle and in conjugation with GPx and GST protects cells against cytotoxicity. So, changes in the dynamics of cancer cell proliferation are accompanied by changes in their intracellular GSH levels that consequently could be reflected in their antioxidant machinery. The present study reported a significant declined level of GSH in cancer control rats compared to normal control rats while the co-treatment of ginger and garlic extract showed an elevated GSH level compared to cancer control rats. The significant elevated expression of Thioredoxins (Trx) and Glutaredoxin (GRx), the key oxidative stress markers in cancer group was due to the increased utilization of these genes for the survival of cancer cells. However, there was a drastic downregulation of TRx, GRx expression in the combined group of ginger and garlic extract in comparison to the cancer group both prophylactically and therapeutically.

The function of inflammation is to eliminate the initial cause of cell injury, clear out the damaged tissues from the inflammatory process, and to initiate tissue repair. During inflammatory responses, the macrophages get activated which release excess amount of various inflammatory mediators such as NO and PGE2 and of pro-inflammatory cytokines such as IL-1ß, IL-6, and TNF-α which are responsible for many chronic inflammatory diseases and cancer. NF-kB is a promoter of inflammatory activities in the body which also regulate proinflammatory genes including IL-1ß, IL-6, and TNF-α. Expression of NF-kB along with the pro-inflammatory markers such as TNF-α, IL-6, IL-10, PGE2 and COX2 revealed a significant upregulation of all the pro-inflammatory markers in cancer group. However, the levels of these pro-inflammatory markers were markedly decreased in the combined group of ginger and garlic extract in comparison to cancer group both prophylactically and therapeutically.

To verify the role of intrinsic and extrinsic pathway involved in the apoptosis, we analyzed the level of Cytochrome c and caspase-9 in the stomach tissue homogenate of experimental animals after 24 weeks of drug treatment. The results infer that ginger and garlic extract in combination significantly improved the level of cytochrome c in cytosol which ultimately activates the caspase-dependent and caspase-independent apoptosis pathway. Simultaneously the level of the anti-apoptotic protein Bcl2 and the proapoptotic protein Bax were determined to characterize the mitochondria mediated apoptosis. Results from this study displayed that apoptosis was mediated by alteration in the level of proapoptotic and anti-apoptotic proteins of Bcl2 family.

Histological analysis confirms the pathological changes in the experimental animals and substantiates the influence of the test drugs. MNU induced cancer control rats divulged non-glandular stomach epithelium which was hypertrophic with vacuolations with focal and atypical glandular hyperplasia. Interestingly, it was noticed that in the non-glandular stomach, epithelium and keratinization was normal in ginger, garlic combination treated rats in comparison to standard drug as well as the individual garlic and ginger treatment group. This clearly confirms the prophylactic and therapeutic protective role of natural foods in elevating the lesion caused due to experimental induction of gastric cancer.

## 5.2 Conclusion

Based on the above study, the prophylactic and therapeutic influence of ginger and garlic extracts together synergistically suppresses the gastric cancer in MNU-induced Albino Wistar rats in a significant manner. The combination of ginger and garlic extract is a potential therapeutic agent to suppress MNU-induced gastric cancer in experimental rats. The probable mode of action of the ginger and garlic extracts in synergism provides a new insight into the chemotherapeutic properties of ginger and garlic, which will allow the design of better management plans for gastric cancer patients. Henceforth, usage of whole extract will be beneficial for the treatment of cancer and its complications rather than its active compounds. The research interest based on ginger and garlic components may provide an approach to decrease the incidence and mortality of gastric cancer. Even though, the free radical scavenging property of *Zingiber officinale and Allium sativum* and its active compounds is found to be almost similar, the anti-oxidant free radical scavenging, anti-inflammatory properties and apoptotic potential shown by the combination dose of *Zingiber officinale and Allium sativum* is found to be superior which will be beneficial in mitigating the several cancer-related complications which are assumed to be majorly caused by oxidative stress. Other than [6]-Gingerol and Alliin, *Zingiber officinale and Allium sativum* contain numerous compounds mediating several biological activities which may synergistically act and may be responsible for its anticancer property. But, the usage of whole extract will be beneficial for the treatment of cancer and its complications rather than its bioactive compounds which will prevent cancer.

## 5.3 Recommendation

This study forms a scientific evidence for the medicinal use of ginger and garlic as anti-cancerous agent and supports its traditional claim by declaring a positive input for a bench to bedside translational research in cancer. Although the results are interesting, further studies are warranted to identify the other mechanisms in mitigating experimentally induced gastric cancers. Subsequently, this could be translated as an adjunct therapy for patients undergoing chemo-radiation therapy. Based on the combination study on ginger and garlic extract for gastric cancer, it is evident that "food is medicine and medicine is food". So, let us all use ginger and garlic paste in our recipes to prevent and mitigate cancer and related disorders. Further studies are warranted to identify if chemotherapeutic agents such as 5-FU can be consumed with ginger and garlic extracts to manage cancer and if it leads to any food-drug interaction.

CPSIA information can be obtained
at www.ICGtesting.com
Printed in the USA
LVHW080325280123
738108LV00014BA/753